TACTICAL FITNESS FOR THE ATHLETE OVER 40

ACTIVELY PURSUING RECOVERY AND HEALTHY MAINTENANCE

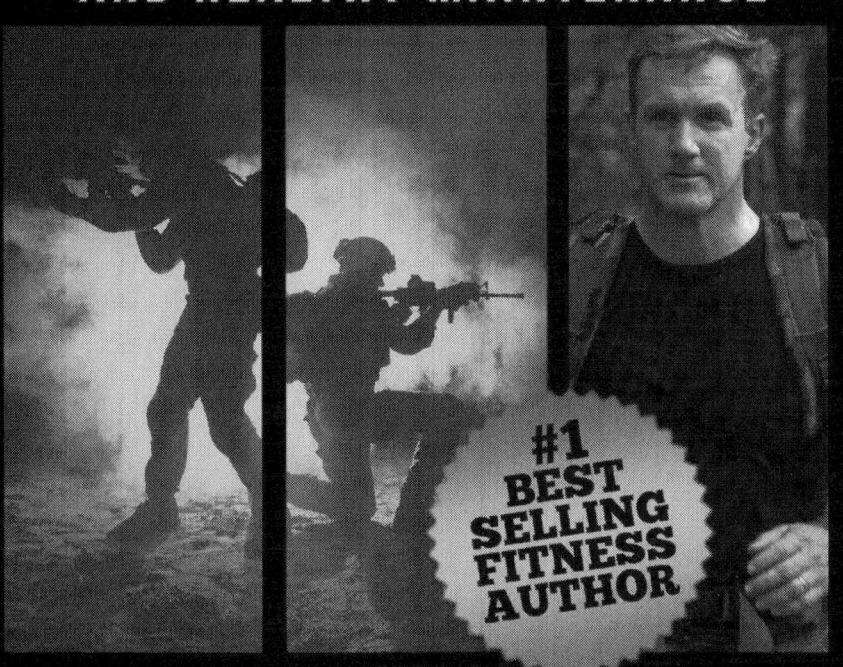

#1 BEST SELLING FITNESS AUTHOR

STEW SMITH, CSCS, USN (SEAL)

ATTENTION:
A Special Note about how this book was created.

Dear Tactical Athlete Over 40,

Thank you for claiming your copy of "Tactical Fitness For the Athlete over 40 - Actively Pursuing Recovery and Healthy Maintenance (An Interview With Stew Smith)"

This book will teach you critical recovery and maintenance skills, tools, techniques and more that every Tactical Athlete Over 40 needs to understand and apply.

This book was originally created as a live interview. Plus, we added exercise pictures, descriptions, links to video, and workouts that focus on all elements of fitness and allows for proper recovery for the tactical athlete.

That's why Section One <u>reads as a conversation</u> rather than a traditional "book" that talks "at" you. However, Section Two and Section Three are more of the traditional fitness book with exercise and workout descriptions / charts.

You can also listen to the video / audio interview if you prefer at the Youtube.com/stew50smith page: <u>Title: *Tactical Fitness Over 40*</u>

I wanted you to feel as though I am talking "with" you, much like a coach or a conversion with a friend AND get a world class workout for the Tactical Athlete Over 40.

I felt that creating the material this way would make it fun for you as we discuss these important topics and put them to use quickly, rather than wading through hundreds of pages.

Get ready to take your tactical fitness training to the next level so you can understand how to train effectively and actively pursue recovery.

Sincerely,

Stew Smith

Stew Smith

Table of Contents

Meet Stew Smith

Published Books Written by Stew Smith

Section One: About Tactical Fitness, Recovery, and Maintenance
Chapter One: Meet Your Tactical Fitness Expert, Stew Smith
Chapter Two: About Tactical Fitness
Chapter Three: Recovery and Maintenance

Section Two: Exercises Descriptions
Chapter Four: Dynamic Stretching and Core Exercises
Chapter Five: Upper Body Calisthenics Exercises
Chapter Six: Dumbbell and Weighted Exercises
Chapter Seven: The Light Weight Shoulder Workout

Section Three: Workouts and Explanations
Chapter Eight: About The Workouts Specifics
Chapter Nine: About Treading and Water Movements
Chapter Ten: The Workout Charts
- Week 1-4: Calisthenics and Weights Transition
- Weeks 5-8: Calisthenics and Running Peak Progressions
- Weeks 9-12: Transition into Weights / Reduce Calisthenics / Running
- Weeks 13-16: Weight Training and Non-Impact Cardio Progression

Closing Remarks

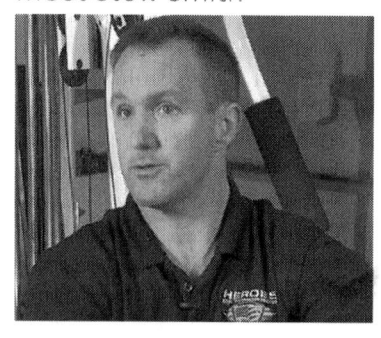

Meet Stew Smith

Stew Smith is an expert in Tactical Fitness training, coaching, and writing whose accomplishments include:

Education:

- US Naval Academy Graduate
- Navy SEAL Training Graduate
- Certified Strength and Conditioning Specialist (CSCS)

Work History:

- Trained thousands of Navy Midshipmen at the Naval Academy
- Trained thousands of military, police, spec ops, and firefighters
- 20+ year history of coaching, training, presenting Tactical Fitness

Awards, Titles, and Designations:

- Amazon Best Selling Fitness Author
- Published Author of Tactical Fitness books and training programs (40)
- Created StewSmith.com 1998
- Created StewSmithFitness.com 2012
- Selling Books since 1998 and eBooks since 2002.
- Online Coaching since 1998

Personal / Business Info:

- Former US Navy SEAL Officer
- Guest instructor at Naval Academy Summer Seminar training 2400 USNA candidates each year for over 20 years.
- Spec Ops Team Coach at the US Naval Academy
- Founder of "Heroes of Tomorrow" which trains military, special ops, police, SWAT, and fire fighters candidates for FREE.
- Created Podcast – Tactical Fitness Report with Stew Smith (Youtube, iTunes, GooglePlay, Soundcloud).
- Full time fitness writer (Military.com, DotDash.com, TheBalance.com) and many other websites and magazines as a freelance writer.
- Works out and writes about it for a living – full time.

Published Books Written by Stew Smith
Tactical Fitness
Tactical Strength - NEW
The Complete Guide to Navy SEAL Fitness
Navy SEAL Weight Training Workout
Maximum Fitness
The SWAT Workout
The Special Operations Workout

General Fitness and Nutritional Guides for Everyone
The Beginner / Intermediate Guide to Fitness
Reclaim Your Life - Erin O'Neill Story (beginner / intermediate)
Veterans Fitness - Baby Boomer and a Flat Stomach!
Circuit Training 101 – Beginner / Intermediate Guide to the Gym
The Busy Executive Workout Routine
The Obstacle Course Workout – Prep for Races or Mil, LE, FF
TRX / Military Style Workouts – Adding TRX to Military Prep Workouts

The Military / Special Ops Physical Fitness Workouts
Advanced Maintenance / Recovery Plan
The Combat Conditioning Workout
Air Force PJ / CCT Workout
The UBRR – Upper Body Round Robin Workout / Spec Ops version
Navy SEAL Workout Phase 1
Navy SEAL Workout Phase 2 - 3
Navy SEAL Workout Phase 4 Grinder PT
Navy SWCC Workout
Army Special Forces / Ranger Workout
Army Air Assault School Workout
Army Airborne Workout
USMC RECON Workout
USMC OCS / TBS Workout
USMC IST and PFT
The Coast Guard Rescue Swimmer / Navy SAR Workout
The Service Academy Workout (West Point, Navy, Air Force Academy)
The Navy, Air Force, Marine Corp Boot Camp Workout
The Army OCS and PFT Workout
Military, Police, Fire Fighter PT Test Survival Guide

The Law Enforcement Physical Fitness Workouts
The FBI Academy Workout | FBI Workout Vol 2
The DEA Workout
The FLETC Workout - Ace the PEB
The PFT Bible: Pushups, Sit-ups, 1.5 Mile Run
The Fire Fighter Workout

Contact Stew Smith (Email, mail)

As part of the downloadable, you do have access to email me at any time and I will answer your questions as soon as possible. Below are the ways to contact me for any of the products and services at www.stewsmith.com.

Mail and email addresses:
StewSmith.com
PO Box 122
Severna Park MD 21146
Email - stew@stewsmith.com

Social Media:

Youtube.com : www.youtube.com/stew50smith (podcasts, swim videos)

Facebook: www.facebook.com/stewsmithfitness (Articles / Q & A)

Instagram: www.instagram.com/stewsmith50 (Cool pics, Motivation)

Twitter: www.twitter.com/stewsmith (Articles, Motivation)

FREE Videos in this Book

In this product, there are free downloadable videos that demonstrate exercises and show techniques in motion by clicking the hyperlinks in the program. These are also on www.youtube.com/stew50smith

© Stew Smith MMXII - All rights reserved. Any part of this book may NOT be reproduced without the permission of the author. Any unauthorized transmission electronic or printed is prohibited.

As with any generic fitness program, this may not be right for you and you should adjust accordingly if needed. Consulting a physician is recommended before undertaking any new fitness program.

Section One: A Conversation About Tactical Fitness, Recovery, and Maintenance

Tactical Fitness Definitions

A quick note on the definition of "tactical athlete" or "tactical fitness". Primarily, the definition is the fitness programming for athletes involved in the military and first responder careers. However, we all should have a certain level of tactical / practical fitness that could help us save our own lives or the lives of our loved ones in the event of a disaster (natural or man-made).

A Conversation with Jim Edwards

Chapter One: Meet Your Tactical Fitness Expert, Stew Smith

Jim Edwards: Hey everyone. And welcome to What's New with Recovery and Maintenance for Tactical Athletes Over Forty, an interview with Stew Smith. My name's Jim Edwards and today I'm talking with tactical fitness expert, Stew Smith, about new developments in recovery and maintenance for the aging athlete **AND** still being able to do physically what you did when you were 20.

Welcome Stew.

Stew Smith: Hey, thanks Jim for having me.

Jim Edwards: Stew is a pioneer in the subject of tactical fitness and has graciously consented to this interview to share extensive knowledge and experiences so every tactical athlete over 40 can learn how to train effectively, avoid injury and recover both mentally and physically from the stresses of the job.

So, my first set of questions is about your background and experience in the field of tactical fitness. Then, we'll jump into your latest ideas and thoughts about recovery and maintenance so our audience can understand how they can apply what you've learned to their situations in today's world.

So, could you tell us a little bit about yourself in terms of background, education and experience in tactical fitness.

Stew Smith: Sure, Jim. As a former SEAL, and a former athlete prior to that, I've had a history of athletics and with that history of athletics comes some good and bad. You develop work ethic, discipline and good habits, but you also build up a history of injuries and even imbalances / weaknesses. But, I am now training people, and have doing so for over 20 years now. These folks want to be in the military, law enforcement, firefighter, and Special Ops professions. I've seen what works, what doesn't work for the tactical athlete. In fact, long before we even called this genre, "tactical fitness", I was writing about it at least a decade before that term existed. We used to call it military, law enforcement, firefighter fitness. I was glad whenever somebody coined the new term.

Jim Edwards: You've been teaching this for 20 years, but when did you get started as an athlete?

Stew Smith: Oh, I was 12 years old I guess, when I first started training but around 8 years old when I started playing organized sports like baseball. We were a big high school football town where I grew up, so everybody started lifting weights in middle school. So, my training days started early in life and I loved it.

And now, I am teaching tactical fitness and learning new ways to recover since I was about 27 years old. Because if you think about it, from 12 to 27, those 15 years can make or break you. And if you go hard and go I mean **hard**, especially into the Special Ops world, you are going to get injured. At 27-28 years old, I was broken. I had to learn how to recover from a life of going too hard. And now at 48 years old, learning and teaching recovery methods is critical to the aging athlete regardless whether you are in the tactical professions or not. In fact, many collegiate level and professional athletes experience the same issues.

Jim Edwards: Is it true that guys in the fire service and other tactical athletes are having to get hip and knee replacements in their 30's?

Stew Smith: Absolutely. I just heard that the other day. I was at a firefighting conference and I met two guys in their 30's who already had replaced hips. It is hard to be an old man in a young man's job. It's hard to be a young man in these professions for that matter.

Jim Edwards: And it's critical that people start learning about this as soon as possible to avoid that type of thing or to mitigate it.

Stew Smith: Oh yes, absolutely.

Chapter Two: About Tactical Fitness

Jim Edwards: So, what kind of things have you done or experiences have you had related to recovery and maintenance that are relevant to our tactical athlete audience over 40?

Stew Smith: You could likely endure decades of training hard and not really need to worry about recovery during your teens and 20's, because let's face it, you just recover faster when you are young. Within 24 hours of a tough workout or day's work, you are ready to go again. But you learn after injury, after injury, after injury, that something is wrong with training hard year-round, year after year. It is best to learn now HOW TO recover and take recovery days even when you are young.

Twenty years ago, I created a periodization program that allows you to grow in all elements of fitness throughout the year, but also allows you to recover from training that has a high chance of injuring you if done continuously year, after year, at high and intense levels.

Even for Spec Ops guy, knowing when and how to pull back, and actively pursue recovery, is critical to your longevity.

Jim Edwards: What roadblocks did you face early on in this area, and how did you overcome them?

Stew Smith: Well, my personal roadblock was just my ego. I'd been going hard for my whole life, and I was a highly active high school athlete. I played a sport every semester I was in high school. In college, I was an athlete and a military student.

Jim Edwards: And you weren't playing wimpy sports either. You were lifting year-round, playing football, then onto college rugby and training to become a better SEAL candidate.

Stew Smith: Yes – we went hard. Football, I still played baseball, wrestled as well. In college, we continued to lift, run hard, swim after practicing rugby, play rugby games – always limping off the field with bumps and bruises. We were doing everything, and year-round doing something.

Stew Smith: Obviously, your body goes through changes from that 12 to 28 years old and the way you worked and played makes a difference on how you feel today. You have a history of traumatic injuries, over-use injuries, muscle imbalances. But there's also some good things like discipline and mental toughness and you build off these habits of fitness that you just can't do without. So, there are good things you learn along this journey. But the mental toughness and discipline can also be your downfall in the end. Your ability to push through your perceived limits, is likely what's going to injure you in the long run. However, this is where things started falling apart for me. After 28 years old, I needed surgery on my ankles, had knee tendonitis annually. Never failed. Every time I ran, I'd get knee tendonitis. Had a stress fracture in my femur. Had a lower back injury. Had a shoulder injury. Things were just falling apart. And I was only 28 years old.

Jim Edwards: And how did that make you feel mentally? Did you just want to keep pushing through it and fighting it and getting passed it for a while?

Stew Smith: It sucked because I am a horrible patient. But, if I had a lower body injury, I still worked out hard just on the upper body and did non-impact cardio. If I couldn't run, I was biking or swimming. I never really stopped unless it was a horrific injury where I just had to stop. Surgery would make you stop. And I remember thinking this would be a good little vacation for me. And then, that's when I realized, if you ever think surgery is a vacation, you might be overdoing it. Think about that. If you ever know somebody who actually says, "Oh, I'll take a break when I get surgery." That's ridiculous.

Jim Edwards: So, you needed to find a better way.

Stew Smith: Yes. Well, I kind of realized then that I was being ridiculous about my training and probably needed to get a little smarter about it.

Jim Edwards: So, do you think that those experiences had anything to do with your current work in recovery and maintenance? Was that what brought you to this point? All those difficult experiences?

Stew Smith: Absolutely. It was purely out of necessity that I started actually creating programs that allowed my body to recover throughout the year but they had to also have a pure focus on the elements of fitness. I went back to my old school, first time ever weight lifting days, and just got back into free and machine weights. And since I couldn't run after surgery. I felt better than I had in years, after cutting out year-round running and just doing some light lifting, some lesser rep calisthenics, spent some time swimming more, and just loosening my body. I couldn't do a whole lot, so I became started stretching and focusing on mobility too. Even learned some yoga.

And this is when I created what I call my solstice running program. If I look back at any one thing that I did, is I figured out a way to adjust my running to look more like a bell curve instead of a flat line up at the top of the intensity level. And it makes sense now. Now, I have a logical progression throughout the year now where I will run harder and do more calisthenics in the spring and summer – peaking there. And then in the fall and winter, I come back down with less mileage and more non-impact cardio and less high rep calisthenics, and more weighted exercises to help rebuild the joints. This process has made all the difference in the world. And that is called, periodization. My way (not THE ONLY way) is just a four-quarter seasonal (12-13 weeks) cycle of training.

Now let me tell you one thing about "periodization". If you type it in Word, it comes up as a misspelled word. If you say, "Siri, what is periodization?" It will come up as ". is Asian." So, nobody knows what periodization is. In fact, every time I give a presentation, I ask, how many of you guys ever heard of periodization? Not many people have ever heard of it.

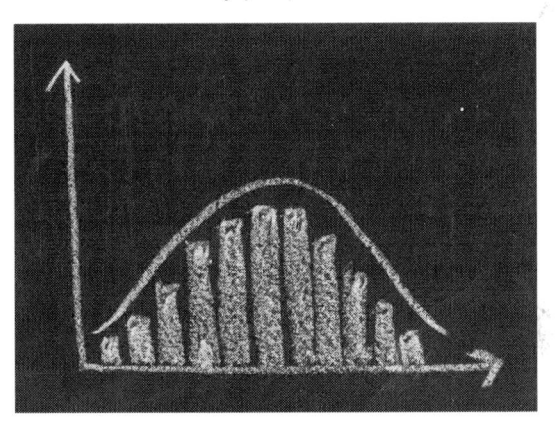

| Jim Edwards: | So, what was your first major breakthrough with recovery and maintenance as a tactical athlete? |

Stew Smith:	Well, periodization! Cycling through all the elements of fitness through the year. You have to think of it kind of like a fitness budget through the year. There are things in your actual budget that you hate paying for, right? What are some of the things you hate paying for in a budget?
Jim Edwards:	Electricity.
Stew Smith:	Electricity, house payment, car payment.
Jim Edwards:	Especially in the summer.
Stew Smith:	And then there's things you love to pay for, like entertainment, restaurants, movies...
Stew Smith:	It is the same way with fitness. There are elements of fitness that we hate to do. Some people hate to run, and they would rather lift. Some people love to run, hate to lift. Some people can't swim. We all have a weakness that we have to work on. And what periodization allows you to do throughout the year, is it allows you to have some fun time with your strengths. But it also allows you to pull in some of your weaknesses so they become less of a weakness.

When I tell people what periodization really is, they have likely done it, they just did not realize it. Typically, it is like before a football season, what did you do? You lifted weights, got strong, ran some sprints. That's preseason training, right? During the season, you probably lifted weights, did some maintenance training, did a lot of practicing. So that's your in-season training. And then post - season, you likely played another sport, or you did some maintenance training with recovery emphasis to nurse any aches and pains. Then you get ready for the next preseason. That's what periodization is. It's just cycles through the year that you are focusing on specific elements. |
| Jim Edwards: | Let me ask you a quick question that's not here, but how do you think periodization affected you mentally or affects others mentally since you know you don't have to do the things you hate at 100%, 12 months out of the year? Does that change your perspective towards your training at all? |
| Stew Smith: | Oh absolutely. It's a break. I've been doing this periodization cycle now for [20 solid years](). Every year, every quarter, I change it up and it is a mental break and obviously, a physical break. Like for instance, right now all my guys and myself are just so excited to get out of the weight room after a winter's hibernation period. And now we're going outside, |

we're running, we're PTing outside, we're in the fresh air. We run obstacle courses. It's just fun and different and a change of pace.

Now, I will say this. By August, early September, we are done running and ready to get back in the weight room.

Stew Smith: It's such a good transition and very refreshing. And it keeps you coming back for more, so you're not skipping workouts. Nothing gets stale. Because a lifetime of fitness is a mental challenge. Every workout you do is a mental challenge. Because you have to get up and go do it. That is mental!

Jim Edwards: As somebody who has been doing this with you now for 4 years, who is well past 40, I can attest to the fact that you are absolutely right. It's about the time you get sick of something, you're on to something else. It's like, hey, we're doing something else and then as you progress, you actually start missing the thing that you disliked before because you're ready to get back to it. And I've seen amazing changes using this as well. So, what Stew's telling you is absolutely 100% the truth.

Stew Smith: Right. Real quick, Jim. We're saying this is for the tactical athlete. But if you think about it, we all should be tactical athletes, right? What do you like to do? You like to shoot guns.

Jim Edwards: I like to shoot guns, do mud runs. I like to play outside with my grandsons, especially when I go to the park. And I'm the only person that's actually playing with the kids, running around and going across the monkey bars and all the old people are sitting there going, who is this fool chasing these children? But I'm having fun and they're all sitting there waiting to die.

Stew Smith: Right. You know, your abilities now, at your age, you are a tactical athlete. Even though you're not a police officer, or a military guy, you are a tactical athlete because you are capable and able to save your grandkids if they were to fall in a river or from other dangers. I won't forget that video you posted of you doing an obstacle during the Spartan Race where I could hear your Grandkids saying, "Good job Grandpa!" I bet there are not many Grandpa's doing Obstacle Course Races.

Jim Edwards:	Right. I could carry somebody out of a burning building if I had to.
Stew Smith:	There you go. That is what I am talking about.
Stew Smith:	When we talk about the tactical athlete, we all could be tactical athletes. Maybe "practical athletes" for lack of a better term.
Jim Edwards:	That's a great distinction. So, how is the world of recovery and maintenance for tactical athletes different now than when you got started? It sounds like it's very different.

Chapter Three: Recovery and Maintenance

Stew Smith:	Yes, the science has evolved a lot. In fact, we are a lot smarter. When I started as a "tactical athlete" as a group, we did not think of ourselves as athletes. And that's the military, police, and firefighters. If at best, we were former athletes, if that makes sense.
Jim Edwards:	Right.
Stew Smith:	There is still much work to be done in that area, because I would say a lot of people in the tactical professions, still don't consider themselves athletes. And I'd say there's been a real big push in the last 10 years to get them to think that way. There was no dynamic stretching used before workouts. The foam roller was not invented yet. The TRX wasn't invented yet. The functional movement screener did not exist, there was no evidence based studies on tactical athletes. All the evidence based science that was out there were on Olympians and professional athletes and college athletes that were trying to break world records. It had nothing to do with recovery of the high stress job, which there's a lot more out there now.
	You know, we've gotten smarter with recovery and over training issues caused by the stresses of the job, nutrition issues, sleep issues, hydration, electrolytes as it applies to the tactical athlete and their performance. Understanding the central nervous system, how it is affected by lack of recovery, stress, injury, rehabilitation, all those things. We are getting a lot smarter with recovery and maintenance of the tactical athlete. When the physiology sciences world joined forces with the tactical world, it made our world much smarter and better. See the Tactical Strength and

Conditioning Journal at the National Strength and Conditioning Association

Jim Edwards:	And do you think people are more receptive to that information instead of just, this is the way it is. This is the way we've always done it. Just shut up and do it.
Stew Smith:	Yes. It really is. And it's been fun watching the genesis of this take off. Like I said, when I first heard the term "tactical fitness", or "tactical athlete", I wrote a book focusing on tactical fitness and we call it, Tactical Fitness. We developed a tactical fitness test that tests every element of fitness, and people are starting to seriously consider themselves as athletes in their job. They see that their fitness level can be the difference between living or dying depending on the situation. Or your fitness can be the difference between you able to save your buddy that's in a life or death situation, or being able to save a victim that you're called to help in your community. Your fitness level can make the difference between someone living or dying. That is how serious we take Tactical Fitness.
Jim Edwards:	And the self-image that comes from defining yourself as a tactical athlete - that is important! But is that something that people have to give up on as they age, or do you believe they don't have to start slowing down at 35 or 40, or 45 or 50. How long do you think people can go for?
Stew Smith:	I've seen people well into their 50's, still doing the same job that they did in their 20's. Now, it does take some luck. And the luck is, not having traumatic injuries along your journey. Now there are some things that just happen to have nothing to do with your training. It could just be an accident, falling through a roof, whatever. Stepping off a truck and breaking your ankle. Those types of things can definitely affect your longevity in these jobs. However, if you stay moderately healthy and away from these traumatic type injuries, or major illnesses, you can definitely stay active well into your 40's and even into your 50's and be the mentor the younger guys need to see - still capable and full of wisdom.
Jim Edwards:	Excellent. Well, it's obvious that you've been around the block when it comes to recovery and maintenance for tactical athletes. Let's switch gears and move into the present where our audience of tactical athletes over 40 specifically, want to know about your latest developments and ideas in this area. What do you mean by, and is it even

	possible to still be able to do physically what you did when you were 20 years old?
Stew Smith:	Is it even possible to be as fit as you were 20 or 30 years ago? I tell you what. Let's do this. Let's take your story.
Jim Edwards:	Okay.
Stew Smith:	What happened to you today?
Jim Edwards:	Today, I called you all excited because I did 20 pull ups in a row and I'm 49 years old. And that was a goal that I set 5 years ago. I could do 20 pull ups in a row when I was 19, and I set this goal when I was 45 and in terrible shape. When I met you and I said, one of my goals is to be able to do 20 pull ups in a row. And today I did 20 pull ups in a row.
Stew Smith:	All right. Hey, congratulations. So yes, as you can see, you did it. You were able to meet your standard that you did when you were 18 years old and probably even 30 or 40 pounds lighter.
Jim Edwards:	No, I weighed 150 pounds when I did it at 19 years old.
Stew Smith:	Right. Well that means you are even stronger now to be able to do that. Because it's a lot more strength involved in doing the pull up at 200 pounds than it is at 150 pounds, obviously.
Stew Smith:	Anyway, there's no reason why at 30, 40, 50+ years of age, we cannot hang with kids who are half our age. It can happen. Now, you won't be world class and beat the best of the best at that young age, but you can definitely hang with the majority and likely stay within a few percentage points of what your best scores ever were in a run, or swim, or even lifts. In fact, many older men are faster and stronger when they are in their late 30's and 40's. Some people even say that you don't even reach your best endurance capacity until you are in your mid 30's. In fact, you can look at like marathon runners and triathlon runners, or triathlon competitors. Some of the best times are usually between 35 and 42. And they're beating the kids that are half their age. Same for strength – old man strength is real!
Jim Edwards:	How do you psychologically, what do you say to the tactical athlete over 40 who is stuck and I have to be able to beat the 18 year olds, I have to be able to beat the 29 year olds. I have to be able to do 30 pull ups or I'm a failure. I have to be able to run a 6 minute miles or I'm a failure. What do you

say to them about balancing the perfect ideal as these alphas tend to do? Because actually just keeping up is a great standard of fitness and you need to just not be so hard on yourself. Does that make sense?

Stew Smith: Mainly the reason why you're able to do this is that you have learned to train properly over the years compared to the new guy who is 20 years your junior. Your experience and knowledge wins nearly every time. Now, will you win every time? Probably not. Will there be events where the young guy is beating you - like a 40-yard dash? Probably. Will you feel tired and a little more banged up 24 hours after a tough workout than the 18-year old? Yes. And that's where the "actively pursuing recovery" term comes in. Whatever you eat and how you sleep and what you drink today to help recover from the workout you just did, helps you to prepare for the workout you do tomorrow. All of these things have to be in perfect balance and taken seriously.

As we age and figure out what works for us best, that's where we get a pretty solid system of what to eat and how to sleep and how to do these little tricks that help us have those little victories. Now, the one thing that you did say was, if I don't get this score, I'm a loser or I'm a failure. You have to take that back half of the sentence out of your vocabulary. Because you're not looking to win every time, or maybe even hit a sub 6-minute mile pace at your age. If you can, that's great. If you can still do 7 or sub 7, that's pretty darned good. And you are still going to beat people in your unit and the younger age group. You might not beat everybody, but you are going to beat some. Now, even if you are the last guy on a run, you give them that, but take them in the pool or get them on pull up bar, or get them on the bench press. There are little victories that you can always rely on that you have.

And I think the alpha guy, that you just said, is a highly competitive soul, and I definitely am one of those guys. If you can train for a little victory every day, it's enough. You don't need to beat all of them. But, as the alpha, as the old guy, you have to also be a mentor to the younger guys and teach them to be you one day.

Jim Edwards: So, how did you actually come up with the idea of recovery and maintenance when it comes to tactical athletes over 40?

Stew Smith: Well, first of all, I am one. I am an aging athlete. I think you have to come to that realization and understand what is happening to you. There are many who are like me who have trained hard all their lives and never stopped training hard. And that's a good thing. However, that also brings baggage and a history of injuries typically. So, this training could also be for those who used to train hard when younger, then took a decade or more off. Kind of like yourself, and you need to rebuild after doctor's reports or a heart attack or scale tips 300 pounds for your first time. These are little warning signs that we have to say, you know what, I can probably up my game a little bit. I used to be hard core. What happened? Then you have to slowly progress back into where you were.

You said it took what, 5 years?

Jim Edwards: Yeah.

Stew Smith: 5 years. Where were you 5 years ago on your pull ups?

Jim Edwards: Oh, I could barely do one. But with work, I saw 5, then 10, then 15 over the years and it kept me motivated seeing progress. I gained pullups as I lost weight (60lbs).

Stew Smith: That's awesome. That is a good progression. And you have to be patient. That's probably the biggest advice I have, is just be patient.

Jim Edwards: So how has periodization and recovery made an impact on your target audience's ability to get results?

Stew Smith: It's made a huge impact. I've been teaching my method of periodization now for over 15 years and I spent five years trying to perfect it. But, I can't tell you how many people email me, text me and say, "I love this periodization program. It's exactly what I needed." What I really like is to hear a 30-year old say, you know what, I felt like I was starting to fall apart a little bit. I didn't have those serious injuries like you did, but I could feel all these symptoms of over training that you mentioned. I felt those coming. I was able to learn from your mistakes and now, at 35, I have no issues and I'm still rolling hard. So, I know it's working really well. And I'm so honored to be able to go and teach it at conferences that appreciated a variety of these periodization programs. Hopefully, one day it will be not just "A" method to train, but maybe the optimal method to train.

Jim Edwards: So, how is what you are teaching better than anything else that's available when it comes to recovery and maintenance for this audience?

Stew Smith: Well, I would say that many of this particular periodization system is my idea. However, I learned a lot much of it from former coaches, school, and from people that are in the business. I get a lot of information from the National Strength and Conditioning Association through their training programs, certifications, conferences. They have some of the smartest trainers in the world at those things. Like I said, I'm honored to go there and teach this system at the Tactical Strength and Conditioning Conferences they have every year. And I usually teach on topics from periodization, recovery, acing the fitness test and mental toughness training to military, SWAT teams, fire fighters, and candidates for these groups.

I would say by people realizing they have to take advantage of recovery methods available, is the biggest thing I teach. People just don't realize they need to actively pursue recovery. That is one of my favorite sayings. Too often, recovery, stretching, warming up / cooling down are neglected by the busy tactical athlete.

Jim Edwards: I can say personally, I've learned that the hard way. If I don't make time for stretching and recovery, then everything goes bad real fast. Why should our over 40 audience switch over to this way of doing or thinking about recovery and maintenance?

Stew Smith: Eventually you will find out that you have to do something different, or you will wind up doing nothing due to your injury history. Plus, this periodization method will teach you not to avoid your weaknesses, like we all have a tendency to do. But we focus on all the elements of fitness and these are: strength, power, endurance, muscle stamina, speed, agility, mobility, flexibility. And if your fitness program right now doesn't include all of those you may want to figure out how you can incorporate them all. They don't have to be all at once or in the same week, these elements and various skills (like swimming, running, rucking) need to be spread out in the course of several months or a year.

Jim Edwards: Okay. So where do you see tactical athletes over 40 wasting a lot of time when it comes to their recovery and maintenance?

Stew Smith:	First of all, it takes time to really add recovery and maintenance. Just because you are stretching after a workout does not mean you are incorporating a recovery session. You need to spend time doing a recovery day. I call mine, the recovery and mobility day (once a week, every other week -.it depends) I typically place in Day 4, which is Thursday in my workout week. My Day 4 Recovery Day start off with a series of dynamic stretches for about 10 minutes, and then I follow that by a variety of non-impact cardio like bike, elliptical, or rowing for about 5 minutes. But every 5 minutes after that, I spend 5 minutes doing foam rolling or stretching combination. I repeat that 5 times. It is a 50 minute "recovery session" workout.

And if you really want to top it off and make it feel even better, go to the swimming pool for about 20 minutes and tread water. You tread water with just your hands and loosen up your elbows and shoulders. You can tread water with just your legs and loosen up your ankles, hips and knees. And then you repeat all the dynamic stretches that you did before you start your workout. You do this in chest deep water. I am sure this quick event alone will help you, especially during the higher mileage running phases that we have in the summer. You can also do this on challenging leg days any time of the year cycle.

But to answer your question, most people do not do this. I would say people are not spending or wasting time doing other things, they are just not adding recovery to their schedule. They are simply neglecting it. |
Jim Edwards:	And part of that is one of your favorite sayings, "If it's not on the schedule, it doesn't get done."
Jim Edwards:	So, if you're going to do recovery and maintenance, you have to schedule the recovery and maintenance as part of your routine. Otherwise, it does not exist or fails to get done.
Stew Smith:	However, be flexible with your schedule. You have to listen to your body. For me, by Day 4 of a hard Monday, Tuesday, Wednesday workout, is the ideal time for me. How about you? What do you need by Day 4?
Jim Edwards:	A break.
Stew Smith:	Face it - some weeks, you feel like crap. And you need to just take an easy day. But, you don't want to skip a workout and do nothing that day. If you want to take a day off, move

	your joints through all ranges of motion, get a little cardio in there, get the heart blood pumping and things will feel better for you. And I promise this Day 4 will make your Day 5 and Day 6 of that workout week so much better than having a hard day 4. That is how you keep rolling.
Jim Edwards:	I'll be honest with you. I look forward to day 4 a lot. Once day 4 is over, I know I can do the next one or two days. I'm a big proponent of Day 4 - Recovery.
Stew Smith:	Yes, absolutely.
Jim Edwards:	Who are the big players in recovery and maintenance that everybody should pay attention to? Who should we be looking to beside yourself?
Stew Smith:	The guys I learned the most from are, I'll just name some of them off the top of my head. You've got Gray Cook, who is a physical therapist. GrayCook.com. He created the Functional Movement Screener (FMS), and it's just a system of basic movements and balancing that test your ability to move your joints properly. Now, where I use it is for myself to see if I am over-training. I can typically pass it. However, when I start to fail a certain exercise in the FMS, like shoulder mobility or the leg lift that tests my balance on one leg, I tend to equate that with, I'm over training. And I need a couple of weeks of mobility days in the schedule to help me balance this out and be able to pass this test. So that's how I Gray Cook's information. He uses it for a variety of other reasons too. But that's a good one for me.

There's another one named Kelly Starrett, and he runs a program called, MobilityWOD. You can go to MobilityWOD.com. And go to his YouTube and see more genius ways to work soreness out of your body. By the way and just Google the following: Functional Movement Screening, MobilityWOD. Also look into the TRX exercises, because Randy Hetrick, who created the TRX Suspension Training Program, is the creator of one of the tools that has probably saved my core and lower back as I have aged. Instead of doing really heavy dead lifts and squats, that tends to compress me these days. Though I still do dead lifts and squats, the TRX is another way to build a very strong core without all the compression that as we age, our discs get thinner and thinner and they can start hurting. Kelly Starrett also wrote a cool book called, The Supple Leopard. It's a great mobility book and it just teaches you |

how to be flexible and mobile with some very innovative and creative ideas.

Stew Smith: How about this one? Some of the tools that we use. For instance, the TRX, foam rollers, lacrosse ball, tennis balls... The foam roller's been out now for a little over 10 years and it's probably changed my life as far as being able to continue running, even with some slight tendonitis flare-ups. It enables you to kind of roll out the pain and roll out the inflammation somewhat to where you're still able to run with less pain, even no pain. But with tendonitis, that pain always comes back when you're not doing anything. But that's when the foam roller can really help. The tennis / lax balls are smaller ways to roll out pain and tight muscles similarly to the foam roller. For more information look into – Myofascial Release.

Jim Edwards: Can I ask a question about foam rollers? Do you have any thoughts about density maybe having a couple different types? Having one that's real dense foam that's hard. Or maybe even like a 6" PVC pipe versus one that might be a little softer or have a softer outside ring?

Stew Smith: The foam roller initially was just a piece of foam, so they were a little more pliable, a little softer. In fact, the more you used them, the softer they got, so you had to get a new one every month if you're really doing it right. And then they started going with a PVC pipe with some rubber wrapped around it, so it added a little bit of cushion, but it stayed rigid. I've had one for two years now, instead of having to buy them every 6 weeks. But yeah, you can definitely use softer ones, harder ones.

In fact, some other mobility tools could be a lacrosse ball. You really want to get into one of those spots on your back or your foot. A tennis ball is a little easier version of the lacrosse ball, used the same way. Also stretching bands. All of those are good to grab onto a limb and help you pull it back a little bit, especially if you can't grab it with your hands. Ice baths, swimming pool. I love running in the water. Whenever I go through my high distance running or hard sprinting, I tend to go to the pool right after the run and swim some laps. But also go in the deep end to tread water and aqua jog. That has been helping a tremendous amount. Treading and doing all your dynamic stretches in the water and the foam rollers, TRX, and straps are really the tools of

	the trade for recovery and maintenance. You can add ice baths if you prefer and that will help with inflammation too.
Jim Edwards:	Well, that pool thing with the ice bath in the summertime actually gives you something to look forward to when you are out running.
Stew Smith:	Yeah. And it feels good. It actually feels like your body is like getting rid of inflammation. As opposed to being out there running and pounding and building inflammation. You will catch a second wind too. By jumping in the pool and reducing your body heat, you will find that perhaps half of your fatigue is due to body heat. So, stay cool or get cool when possible!
Jim Edwards:	There you go. What are the big challenges for tactical athletes over 40 when it comes to recovery and maintenance right now?
Stew Smith:	Depending upon the seriousness of your previous injury history, stretching and range of motion exercises can be rather challenging at first. But, with patience and belief that you need to take a recovery day off from a hard training week, you will see the results and feel better in general.
Jim Edwards:	Excellent. So, is this the end of the road of your journey, or are you still making new discoveries to help people with recovery and maintenance?
Stew Smith:	First – fitness IS a journey – not a destination. I tell people that we should ALL be on a constant search for recovery tools of the trade and education. Experiment with different programs, even supplements that claim better recovery after using, but figure out what works for you. I found some additional protein each day can help with recovery (food or powder form). That has probably been my biggest noticeable improvement compared to a large variety of supplements you can put into your body.
	I prefer food and protein powders that ARE food. And they are food if they say Nutritional Facts on the back of the label. I don't know if you've ever noticed that, but you ever look, check out a package of vitamins and supplements. The ones that are actual food say "Nutritional Facts" and the ones that are supplements, say "Supplement Facts". And supplements really can be a variety of ingredients that you may or may not even need. Some supplements may not be helpful to you at all and you are likely wasting your money.

You have to remember that supplements are not regulated by the Food and Drug Administration for their claims that they make. You never know. They could be harmful for you as well or at do nothing. I personally like this natural whey protein from Ascent.

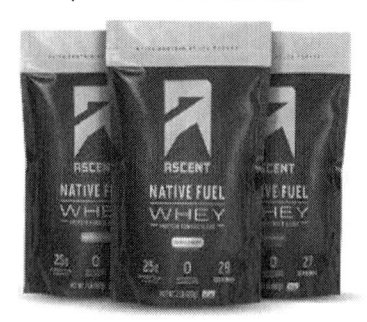

Whey Protein - Native Whey Produced!

Jim Edwards: What short or long term developments do you see on the horizon for this area? What do you see coming down the road for all this?

Stew Smith: Well, the one thing I don't see is a magic pill that is going to be created that will make us recover better and be more mobile. So, it takes time and patience and focus. Like I said, you have to actively pursue recovery in order for it to work for you. You also have to keep an open mind and try new things as they develop.

I found what works for me, and it may be great for you as well, or you may prefer other recovery tools or methods like yoga class, meditation, or doing a spin class, if you like that kind of group training. Paddle boarding, something that's relaxing and fun. Find a non-impact cardio activity that you enjoy. Relax through full range of motion exercises. Even then, if you think you know it all, you need to still keep an open mind and try to see what's new out there. Because it may be the best thing ever for you. I personally find that running every OTHER day really helps me now in my late 40's. In fact, I have the program in this book as a running every OTHER day option with a tough non-impact cardio day in between OR a cardio / mobility day in between tougher workout days. If you need to you can opt out and run daily if you are not hurting from previous running days.

Jim Edwards: So what haven't I asked you about recovery, maintenance, and periodization? Any final thoughts do you have that might help motivate people in this area?

Stew Smith: You know the main thing I'd like to add to this is check out the workout weeks in this program. They are going to be a combination of cardio, resistance, mobility, active recovery days and NOT EASY. Sometimes a picture of a week of training is worth a thousand words, so what I'm doing in the next chapter is creating a picture and descriptions of the exercises and four by four week cycles that represent each one of the periodization phases. You have a Spring run progression with calisthenics and some lifting combinations. You have a Summer run max and calisthenics maximum. You have a Fall where you still run but a little bit less. This transition involves more swimming or other non-impact cardio activities and you tend to have a 50/50 split of calisthenics and lifting. And then the Winter is a pure lifting cycle with some non-impact cardio. All phases require some mobility days off. Mobility / Recovery are also arranged in there and you can actually pursue recovery from previously challenging cycles.

Enjoy the (4 x 4 weeks) 16 week training program for the aging tactical athlete as an example of what you can do as you age. But even before your inevitable overuse injuries, start mixing in mobility and recovery days now. Even when you're young. Because even though you're still in your 20's, and you don't feel like you need to recover, guess what? You need to recover and start learning how to recover. Some people even say this, and I'm not quite into this mentality yet, however, they say" if you're in your 20's, you need to train like you're in your 30's. If you're in your 30's, you need to train like you're in your 40's. If you're in your 40's, you need to train like you're in your 50's". I can't say I've taken to that mentality, but I understand what they mean. Because there are days when you need to train like you are older in order to one day be older and still have the same abilities that you have now.

Jim Edwards: One of the things that I'm getting from you on this, and I hope I'm not overstepping my bounds, but it sounds to me like old age and your history are going to win out over youthful enthusiasm in this, and we have to have a lot more planning, being much more thoughtful, much more strategic in how we train, and the methods that we use to recover so that we can keep going. You can't just go out and perform

	like when you were 18 or 20 and can recover naturally the next day. You need to have a plan in place and a strategy to keep yourself mobile and recovering on a regular basis. And that's really the crux of all of this as it takes proper planning and education and understanding if you want to remain successful as a tactical athlete as you age.
Stew Smith:	Absolutely. And, you know, you need to check your ego at the door a little bit. And that's hard. It's hard for me to do every day. But there will be a day when I realize that I am probably going to have to do more yoga based exercises and swimming. And those will be my resistance and cardio days. Hopefully, I can still be able to lift with healthy joints that don't ache, but there may be a day when that is not going to happen.
	But you never know. I just watched TV the other day and watched a 90 year old guy lifting weights in the weight room. As one thing I've always done, is I remember when I was 20 and there were 50-year old SEALS that were working out with us. And I remember saying, "when I'm his age, I want to be like him." I am now the age of the guy I wanted to be when I was 22. It can happen. You just have to get smart about it. And eventually I got smart about it.
Jim Edwards:	Awesome. So, how would you sum up everything that we've discussed today in a few final thoughts and advice to our listeners and readers?
Stew Smith:	You know what? I would say this. I'm a fitness writer. I've been working and writing about periodization for years now.
	One option is the Maximum Fitness book - It was an advanced 52-week training cycle with all four quarters (4 x 13 week cycles) focusing on all the elements of fitness spread throughout the year. Also, the book, Tactical Fitness is a very challenging program and a little more advanced level. But it tests all the elements of fitness in what is called the Dirty Dozen Tactical Fitness Test. It has workouts for your upper body, lower body, full body, cardio, and core applied in a tactical testing format. The books focus on all the elements of fitness: strength, power, muscle stamina, speed, agility, endurance, mobility and flexibility arranged throughout the year so you do not burnout on any one element of fitness.
	If you want to stay strong, keep lifting. The Tactical Strength book, is a pure lifting, speed / agility with moderate cardio

cycle (plenty of non-impact options) that focuses primarily on strength and power. It has some faster cardio (speed and agility) with limited impact cardio.

Of course, there are many free articles out there that you can read about how we implement periodization and mobility into training year-round. If you want to read more about periodization and designs to help you recover, improve performance, and build a body for longevity, check out the related articles from the Military.com Fitness Archives:

More about Periodization
Periodization Training
Periodization – Do I Need It?
Periodization Advice
Multi-Sport Athlete Periodization
Summer – Fall Transition

Jim Edwards:	Tell people about your PT club. How you and I met. How people can work with you one on one.
Stew Smith:	I also do online coaching. It is really for anybody who may not like to alter programs and books to suit their needs, I do that for you. We work one on one together and I send you weekly workouts for you and your feedback helps me create the following week and we just keep going through week after week, after week until you say all right, I think I'm done. And most people don't ever leave. I have had people on here like Jim, for over 5 years and I think I have another guy that just hit like 300weeks of workouts. Over 6 years.
Stew Smith:	It's also a lot of fun. It's a 12 week program that you just keep reusing every 12 weeks if you want, or you can get new stuff every 12 weeks. It depends on your goals and your desires or what you want to do with your fitness performance.
Jim Edwards:	And I highly recommend it if you're serious about being a tactical athlete, or operating at the level of a tactical athlete, Stew Smith can help you tremendously. Thanks very much for sharing your expertise and experiences so graciously. And thank you to all the tactical athletes over 40 in our audience for your service and joining us for this presentation about you can get better results with recovery and maintenance and how to train effectively and actively pursue recovery. Have a great day.

Section Two: Exercises Descriptions

Getting Started

The following stretching plan will assist you with getting started again safely and without as much post-exercise soreness.

Most injuries are strains or muscle pulls that can be prevented with a few simple stretching exercises done daily. The added flexibility will not only assist in injury prevention, but with speed workouts and help you to run faster. The following is a stretching routine that can be used whether you are a beginner or advanced athlete.

The Warm-Up Routine

Finding what works best for you as a warm-up is critical to your success in either fitness testing as well as long term job performance. Increasing your flexibility should be the first goal before starting fitness/athletic activity. This dynamic stretch routine is a quick and effective way to warm up prior to your workout as well as cooldown in the pool afterwards to produce the desired results of mobility and flexibility.

Chapter Four: Dynamic Stretching and Core Exercises

A quick and easy to follow dynamic stretching routine will demonstrate the way to warm up and prepare for workouts. Take 5-10 minutes and get warmed up with these leg movements prior to working out. You can do this one land (typically) or add a session in chest deep water. Click the hyper link to see most of these in motion.

- Jog or Bike - 5 minutes
- Butt Kickers - 1 minute
- Frankenstein Walks - 1 minute
- Bounding in Place - 1 minute
- Side Steps with hip opener – 1 min
- Leg Swings Front / Back– 1 minute
- Leg Swings (Left / Right) – 1 minute
- Calf/Shin Warm-up – 1 minute
- Burpees – 1 minute
- Light Arm Shoulder Chest Stretch
- Light Thigh Stretch
- Light Hamstring Stretch
- Back Roll
- Light ITB Roll
- Shin Roll

Warming Up / Cooling Down for Workouts

Jog five minutes or do a series of light calisthenics like jumping jacks, crunches, push-ups, squats prior to stretching. Dynamic stretching is a major part of warming up prior to any athletic movements. In order to reduce muscle fatigue and soreness and perhaps prevent injuries, perform a good warm-up using these dynamic/static stretches. You can also use these on the back end of a hard workout to cool-down from hard activity. Perform in the pool for even better results as a cool down.

Jog or Bike 5 minutes – Get the blood flowing.

<u>Butt Kickers</u> - **1 minute:** Jog slowly and flex your hamstrings to pull your heels to your butt on each step. Do with knees down and knees up for 30-60 seconds.

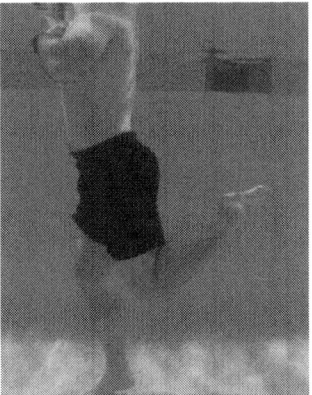

<u>Frankenstein Walks</u> - **1 minute:** Walk and kick high each step. Try to kick your hands in front of you. Do 10 kicks with each leg.

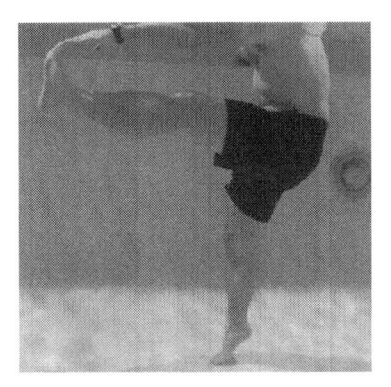

<u>Bounding</u> - **1 minute:** Do high powered skipping for 1 minute. Start off with regular skipping then lift knees high each step. Do in place for 1 minute

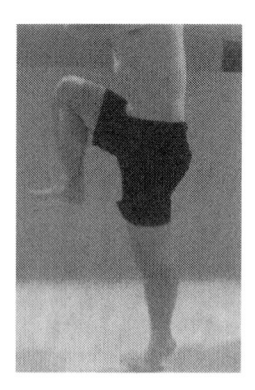

<u>Side steps w / hips openers</u> - **30 seconds each direction:** Work lateral movement into the warm-up. Step sideways by lifting the leg and opening the hip to the side you step. Do for 1 minute back and forth alternating in each direction.

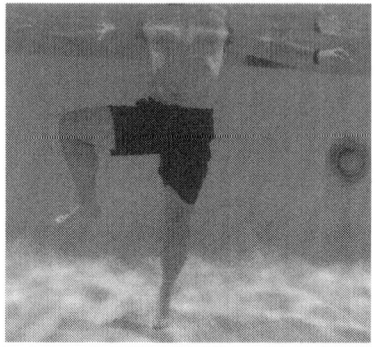

<u>Leg swings</u> – **1 minute:** Stand still and lift legs back and forth with legs straight at full range of motion of your hip (front / back). Then swing leg left and right in front of your body for 10 reps each leg.

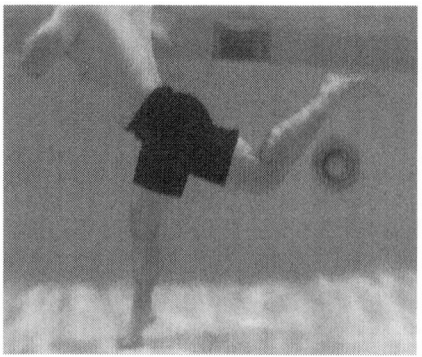

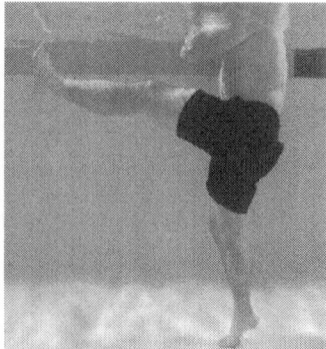

<u>Side Leg swings</u> – **1 minute:** Stand still and lift legs back and forth with legs straight at full range of motion of your hip side to side (left / right).

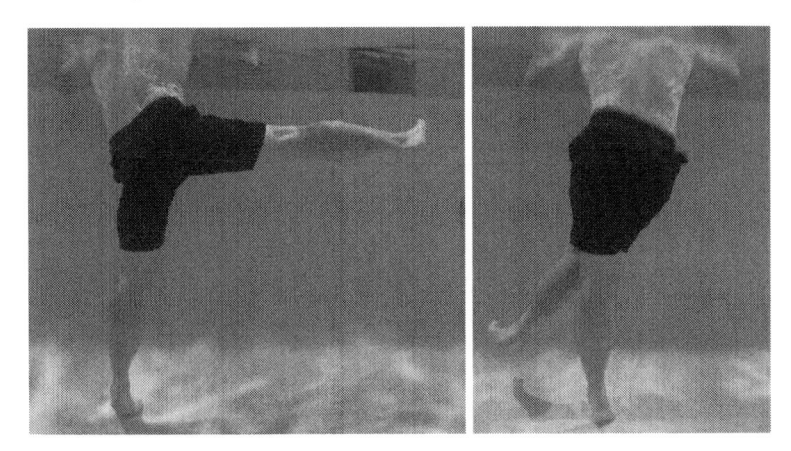

Calf/Shin Warm-up – 1 minute: Alternate lifting heels off the floor and toes off the floor. This is a shins/calves builder to help strengthen legs for running/rucking.

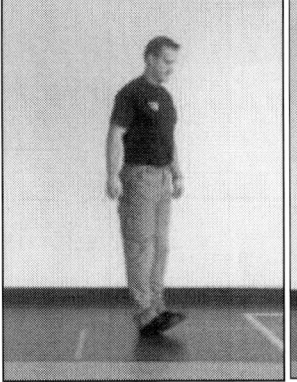

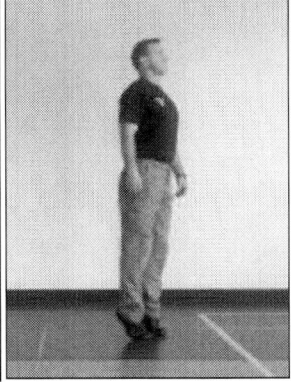

Burpees – 1 minute: Drop into the pushup position. Quickly drop your chest to the floor and back to the up position. Bring your feet up and stand and jump 4-6" off the ground to finish the rep.

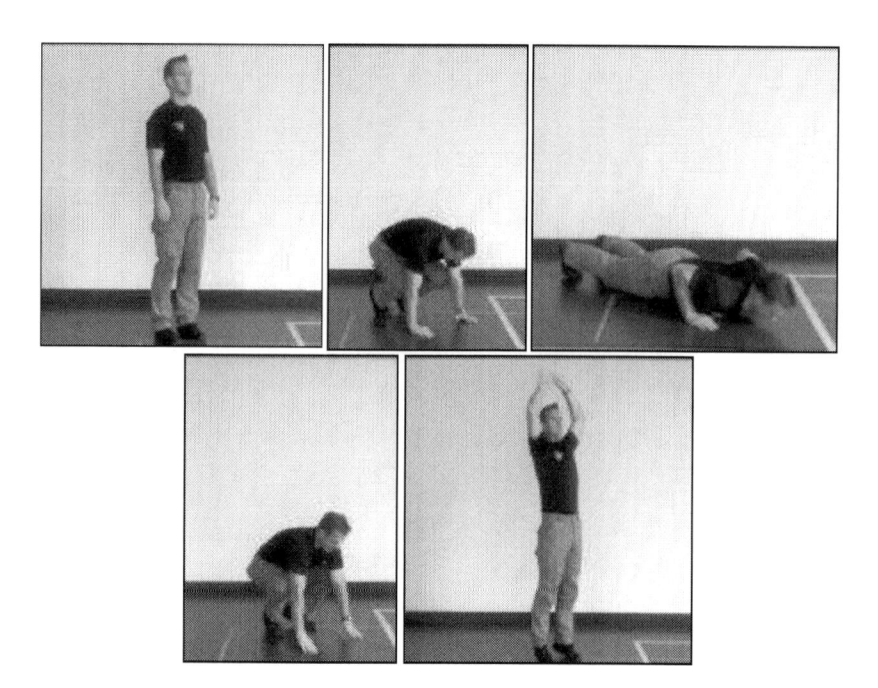

Light Arm Shoulder/Chest stretch: Pull your arm across your torso to stretch rear/deltoid and trapezius region. Then pull your arms backward as far as you can to stretch the chest/front shoulder connections.

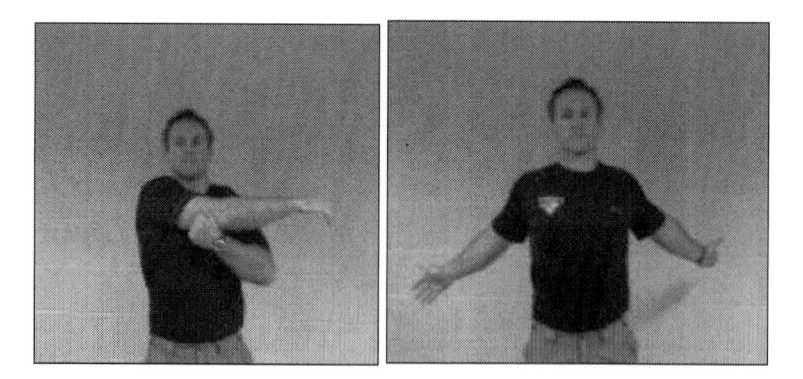

Thigh Stretch – Standing: - Standing, bend your knee and grab your foot at the ankle. Pull your heel to your butt and push your hips forward. Hold for 10-15 seconds and repeat with the other leg.

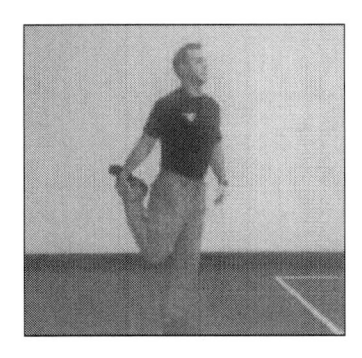

Hamstring Stretch #1: - From the standing position, bend forward at the waist and come close to touching your toes, slightly bend your knees.   Go back and forth from straight legs to bent knees to feel the top/bottom part of the hamstring stretch. You should feel this stretching the back of your thighs.

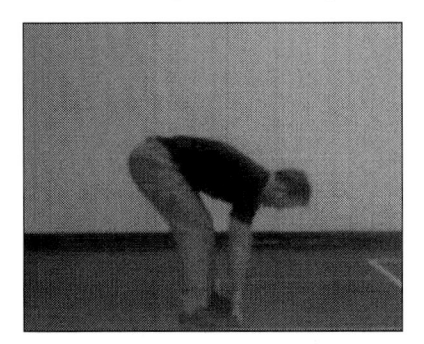

More Stretching Plans

There is a supplemental stretching plan full of exercises that can be found in the lower back plan (legs, hips, core). In an effort to save space, for pictures of static stretches, check out the PDF file:

Lower Back Plan

http://site.stewsmithptclub.com/lowerbackplan.pdf

Foam Rolling - **Myofascial Release** Foam Roller Article / Video

Back roll: Sit on foam roller and move slowly back and forth as you lie on the roller. Move your legs to move your body over the roller. Do for 1-2 minutes each body part.

ITB roll: Lay on your side in a side plank position and place foam roller under your hip. Move forward and roll your ITB from the hip to below the knee. Do for 1-2 minutes on each side of the leg.

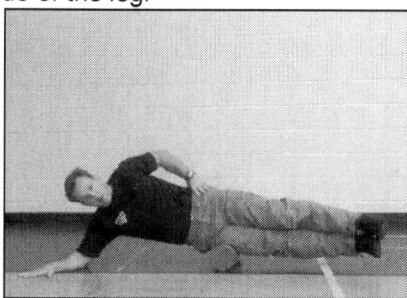

Shin Roll: Place roller under your knees and slowly kneel down placing both shins on the roller. Slowly roll back and forth from bottom on the knee to the top of the ankle.

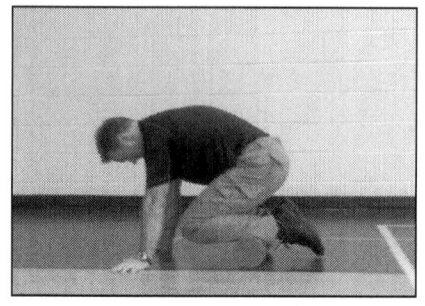

Core Workout Exercises

Abdominal exercises as a warm up before/after stretching

When you exercise your stomach muscles, make sure to exercise and stretch your back also. The stomach and lower back muscles are opposing muscle groups and if one is much stronger than the other, you can injure the weaker muscle group easily.

Advanced Crunch - **(Legs up):** Lie on your back with your feet straight in the air. Keep your legs straight up in the air for the advanced crunches. Cross your hands over your chest and bring your elbows to your knees by flexing your stomach.

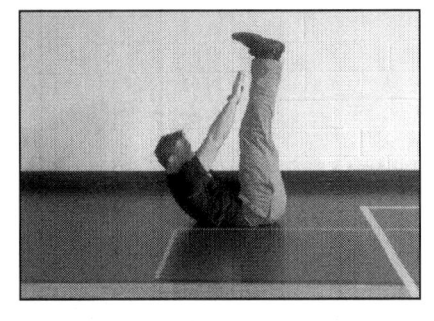

Reverse Crunch: In the same position as the regular crunch, lift your knees and butt toward your elbows. Leave your head and upper body flat on the ground. Only move your legs and butt.

(Do not do if you have severe lower back injury or if this hurts your back)

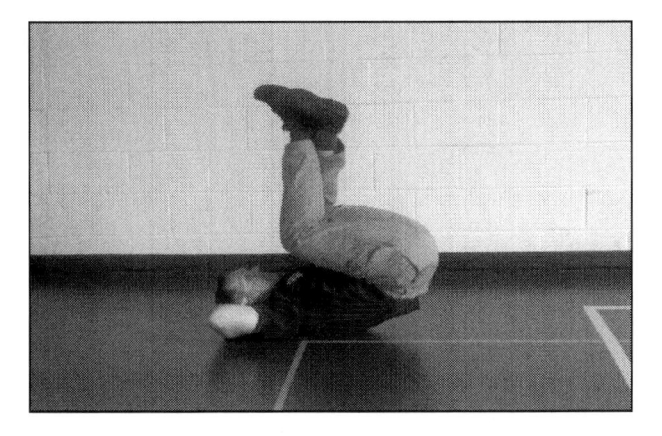

Double Crunch: Lift hips and shoulders off the floor at the same time in one motion.

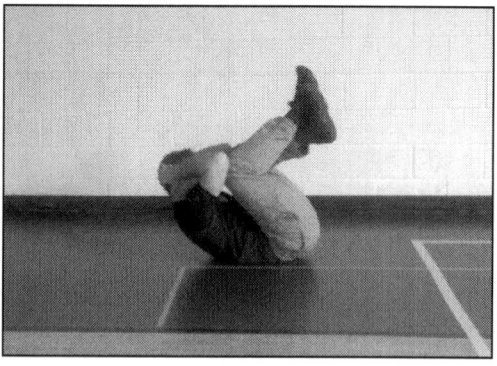

Right Elbow to Left Knee: Cross your left leg over your right leg. Flex your stomach and twist to bring your right elbow to your left knee.

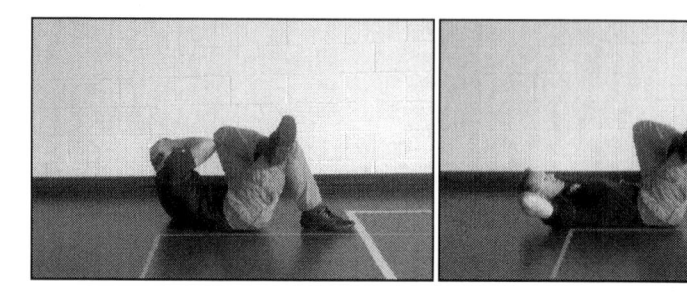

Left Elbow to Right Knee: Cross your right leg over your leg. Flex your stomach and twist to bring your left elbow to your right knee.

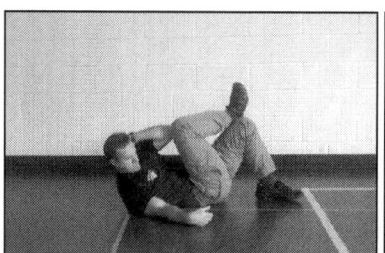

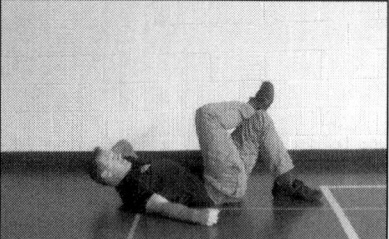

Bicycles: This is a mix between opposite elbow to knee crunches with bicycling of your legs. Alternate from side to side for prescribed reps and do not let feet touch the floor.

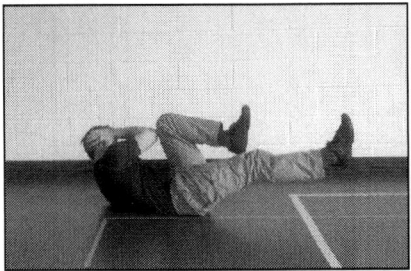

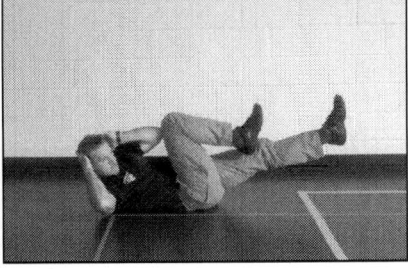

Sit-ups: Lie on your back with your arms crossed over your chest, or hand locked behind your head (Army / FBI Style) keeping your knees slightly bent. Raise your upper body off the floor by contracting your abdominal muscles. Touch your elbows to your thighs and repeat.

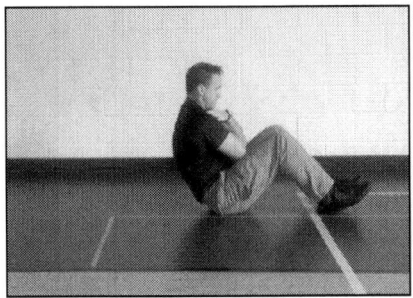

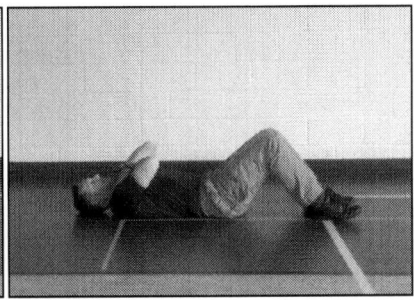

Lower Back Exercise - Swimmers: Lie on your stomach and lift your feet and knees off the floor by flutter kicking repeatedly as if you were swimming freestyle – build up to 1:00 – or keep feet still but off the floor.

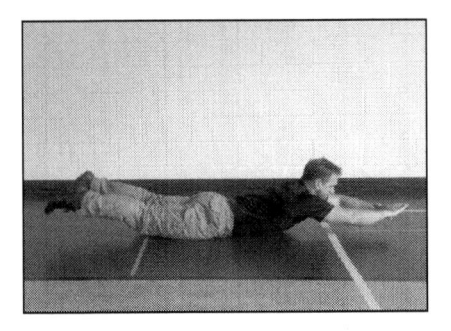

Lower Back Exercise #2 - Hip Rolls: Lie flat on your back with your knees in the air as in the middle picture below. Keep your shoulders on the floor, rotate your hips and legs to the left and right as shown below.

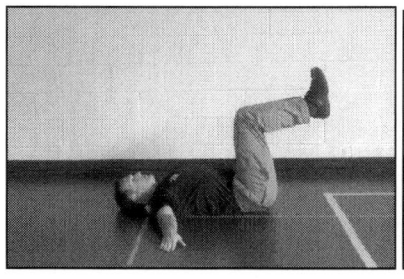

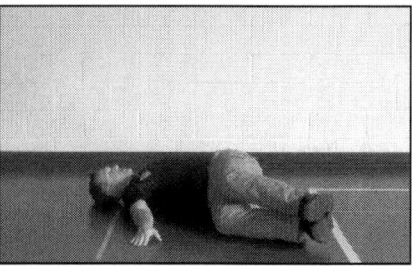

Upper back exercise #1 - Arm Haulers: Lie on your stomach. Lift your chest slightly off the floor and wave your arms from your sides to over your head for 30 seconds.

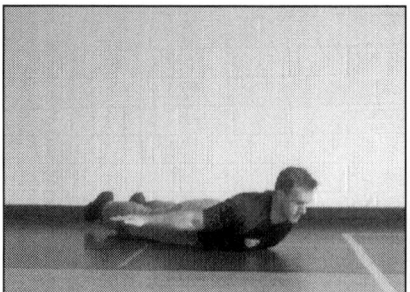

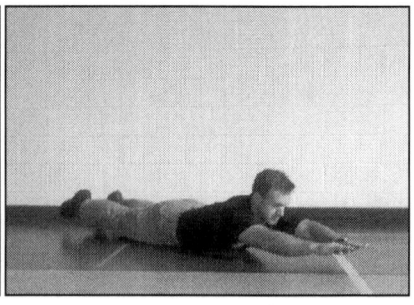

Upper back exercise #2 - Reverse Push-ups - Lie on your stomach in the down push-up position. Lift your hands off the floor instead of pushing the floor. This will strengthen your upper back muscles that oppose the chest muscles.

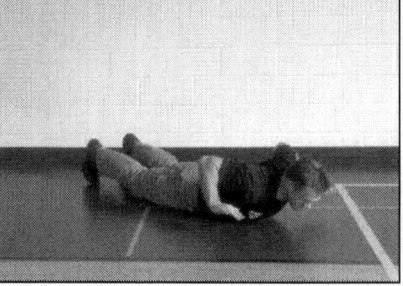

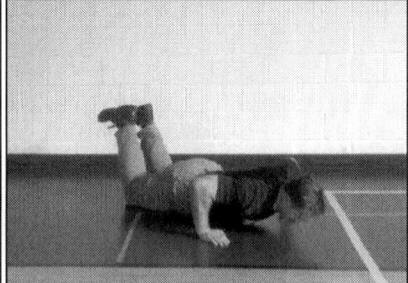

Upper back exercise #3 – Birds: Lie on your stomach with your arms spread to the height of your shoulders. Lift both arms off the floor until your shoulder blades "pinch" and place them slowly in the down position. Repeat for 10-15 repetitions mimicking a bird flying.

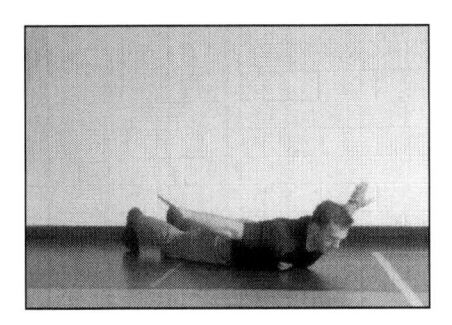

Plank Pose and One Arm Plank: To complete the Crunch Cycle, try getting into the plank position and see if you can hold it for at least 1 minute. As you advance, lean on the left / right arm as you increase the time. Or do the plank in the UP Pushup position.

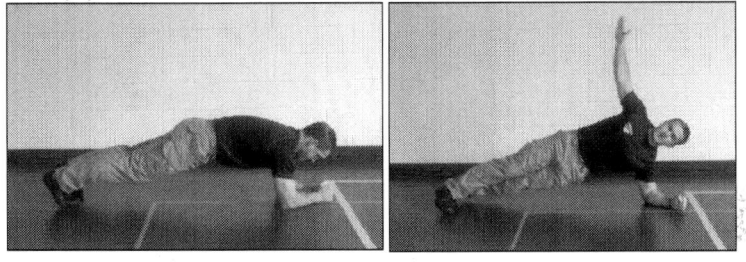

In fact, when you fail at pushups during the workout, stay in the UP Pushup position for an extra 30-60 seconds each time. This will prepare you well for the long periods of time in the "leaning rest" as well as strengthen the core for crawling obstacles.

Bear Crawls – Walk like a bear on all fours. This gets tough after a couple hundred yards. (crawling benefits)

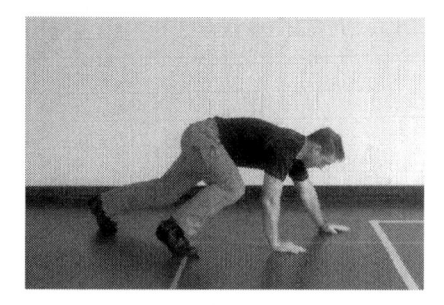

Tip to reduce strain on the lower back WITH LEG LEVERS and FLUTTERKICKS - Lift your butt off the ground about an inch and place your hands underneath your butt bone, thus taking some of the strain off the lower back.

Flutter-kicks - Place your hands under your hips. Lift your legs 6 inches off the floor and begin walking, raising each leg approximately 36 inches off the ground. Keep your legs straight and moving. This is a four count exercise.

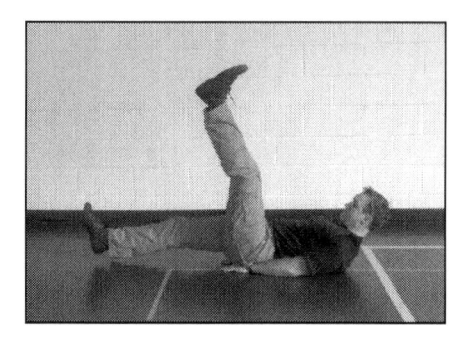

Leg levers - Lift your feet 6 inches off the floor. Raising both legs approximately 36 inches off the ground, keep your legs straight and off the floor until specified number of repetitions are complete.

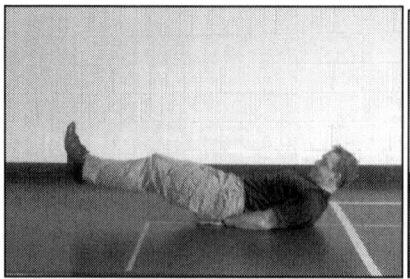

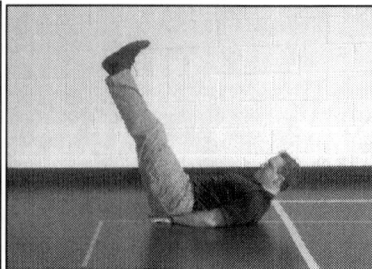

Chapter Five: Upper Body Calisthenics Exercises

Regular Push-ups - Lie on the ground with your hands placed flat next to your chest. Your hands should be about shoulder width apart. Push yourself up by straightening your arms and keeping your back stiff. Look forward as you perform this exercise. *(You can also mix in wide and close stance pushups for variety if you prefer.)*

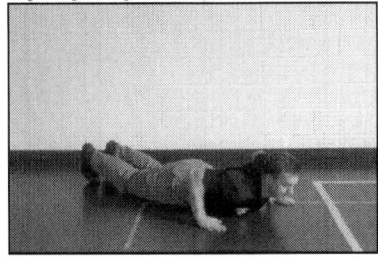

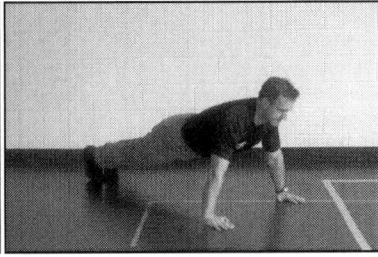

Parallel Bar dips - Grab the bars with your hands and put all of your weight on your arms and shoulders. Do not do these exercises with added weight, if you are a beginner, or if you have had a previous shoulder injury. **To complete the exercise, bring yourself down so your elbows form a 90 degree angle (no less of an angle) and back to the up position.**

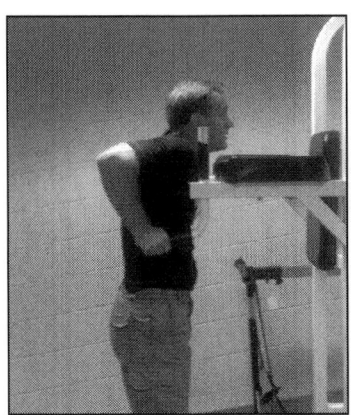

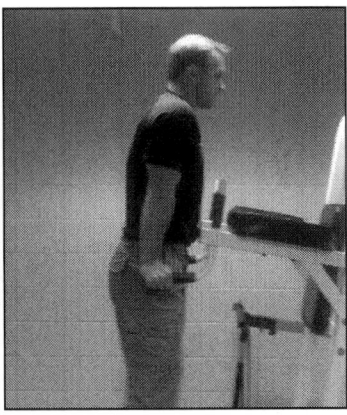

Get good at pull-ups and dips as they will help you pull yourself up and over climbing obstacles when faced with a wall, rope, or ladder climb

8 Count body builder push-ups - The all-time favorite group PT exercise and ideal for preparing for an obstacle course as a great simulation exercise when mixed with pull-ups and short runs / crawls etc…

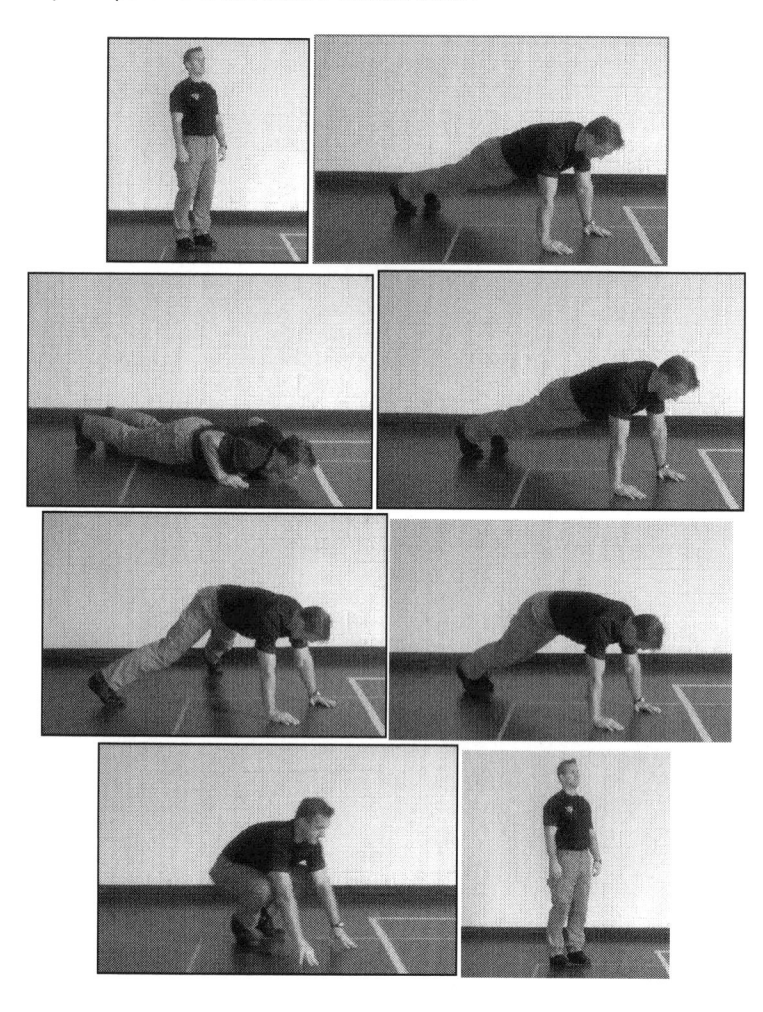

Pull-ups (regular grip) - Grab the pull-up bar with your hands placed about shoulder width apart and your palms facing away from you. Pull yourself upward until your chin is over the bar and complete the exercise by slowly moving to the hanging position.

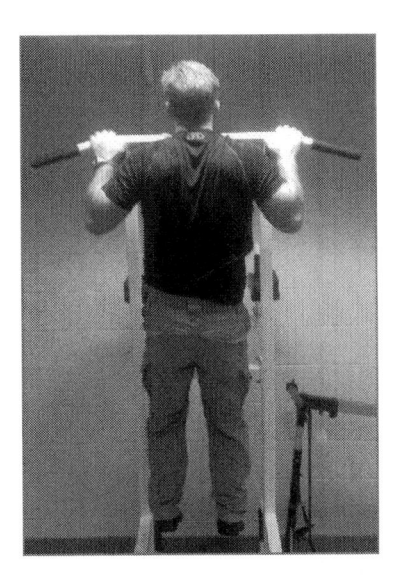

Mix in different grips for a variety (wide grip, close grip, alternated grip)
*Note – When using a reverse grip - keep your hands in and do not go wider than your shoulders as you will develop some elbow tendonitis similar to that of tennis elbow.

When you fail at pullups, add in DB rows or pulldowns to complete the set

Squats - Keep your feet shoulder width apart. Drop your butt back as though sitting in a chair. Concentrate on squeezing your glutes in your upward motion. Keep your heels on the ground and knees over your ankles. Your shins should be near vertical at all times. Extend your buttocks backward. Do with or without a dumbbell / kettlebell in your hands.

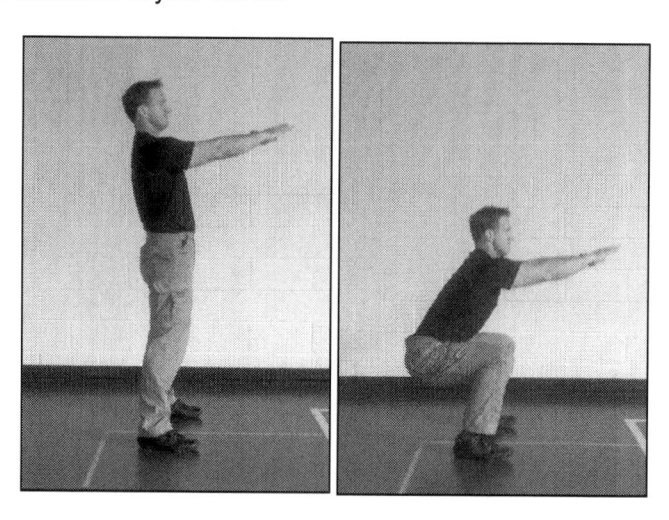

Walking Lunge - Keep your chest up high and your stomach tight. Take a long step forward and drop your back knee toward the ground. Stand up on your forward leg, bringing your feet together and repeat with the other leg. Make sure your knee never extends past your foot. Keep your shin vertical in other words.

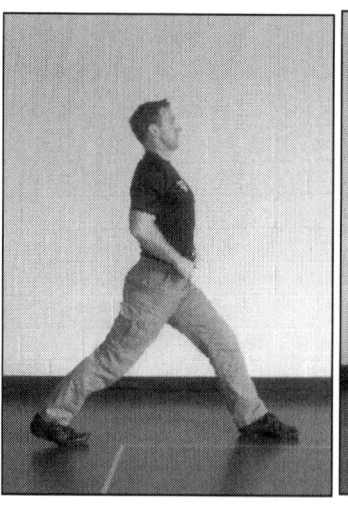

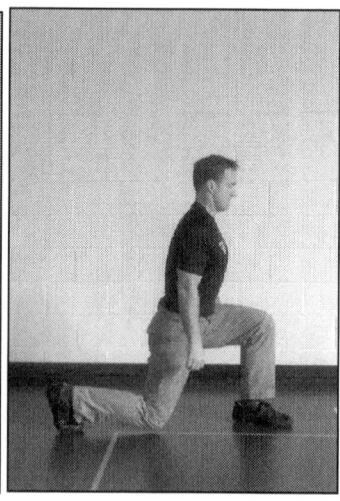

Box jump - 20 inches universal height – straighten torso / hips for complete repetition. Step or jump down and repeat. As you age, you may prefer to step down instead of jumping.

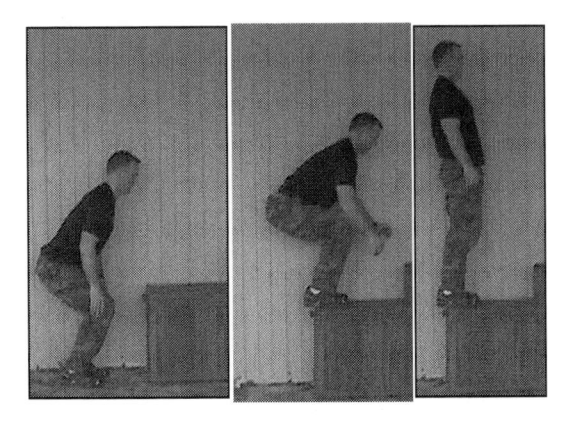

Stair Crawls – Here is an upgrade on the bear crawl. Crawl head first down the steps and feet first UP the steps for a challenging core and shoulder girdle workout.

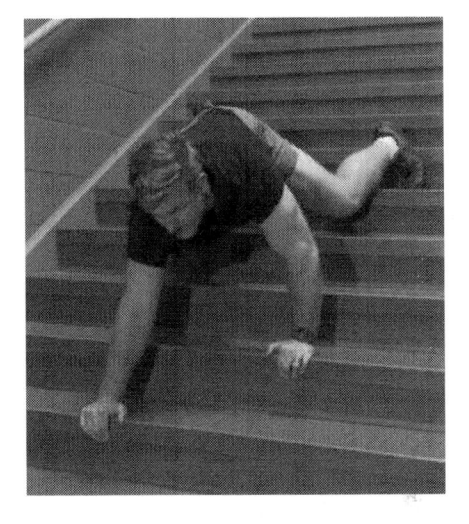

Chapter Six: Dumbbell and Weighted Exercises

Bench Press: Lie on your back on a bench, placing the legs bent with feet flat on the floor on both sides of the bench. Extend your arms upward, grab the machine, barbell, or dumbbells just greater than shoulder width and lower the bar to your chest slowly. The bar should hit just below the nipples on your sternum. Extend your arms again to a locked position and repeat several times.

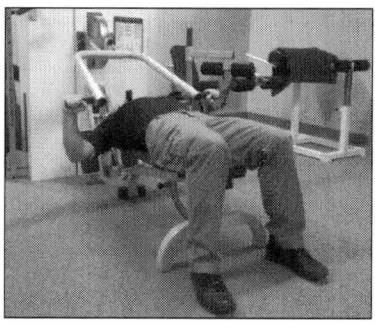

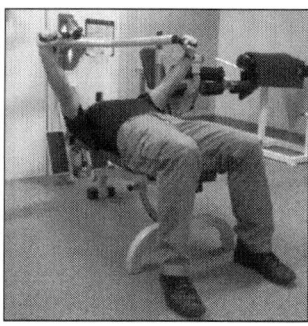

Pull-down Machine – This is an easier form of pull-ups, but you have to start somewhere. Using a pull-down machine, grab the bar, sit down and pull the bar to your collar bones. Keep the bar in front of you. Keep the bar moving in front of your body / not behind your head. **Change grips as you can on the pull-up bar (wide, regular, close and reverse).**

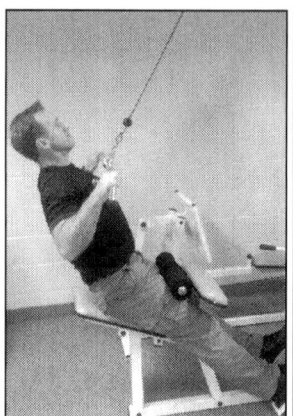

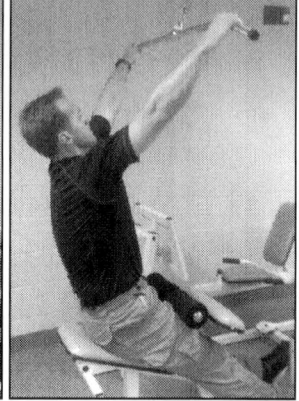

DB rows – Grab dumbbell (DB) in one hand and lean forward onto a bench supporting your back with your opposite knee and hand on the bench. Pull the DB up to your chest, hold for 1 second and slowly extend arm. Repeat 10/arm.

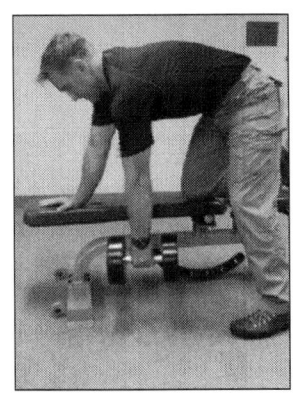

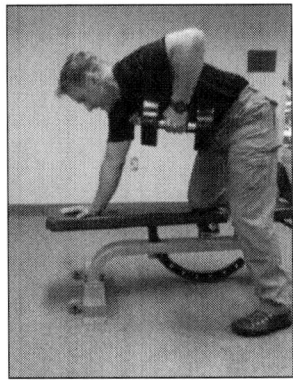

Wood Chopper Squat with Dumbbell – Add a dumbbell to the squat by swinging the weight over your head when standing and between your legs when squatting. Keep head up and back straight.

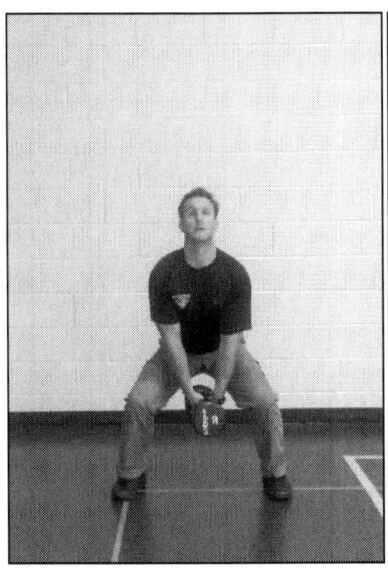

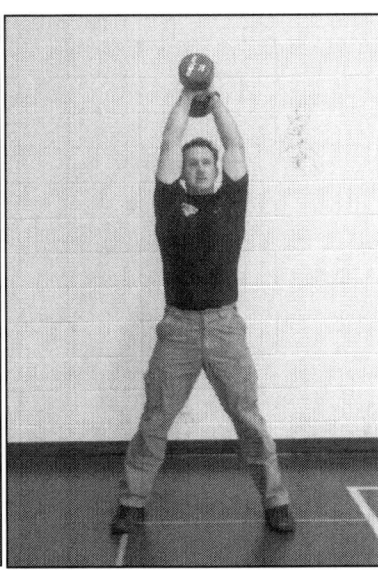

Kettle bell swing – Similar to the woodchopper squat, explode with your legs and hips to get the kettlebell or dumbbell above your head.

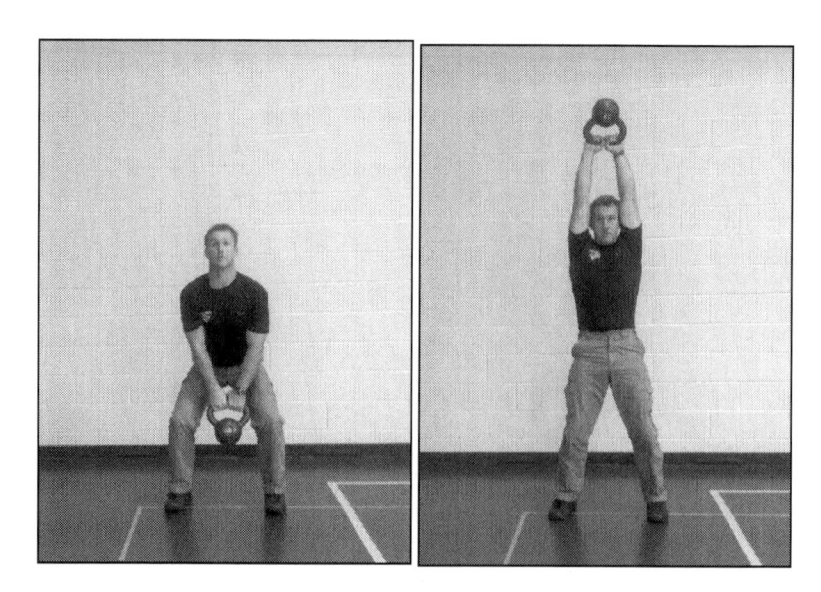

MJDB #1 - Multi-Joint Dumbbell Exercise: Perform a bicep curl, then press the dumbbells over your head with a military press, and then go straight into a triceps extension - repeat in reverse order to get to the starting position.

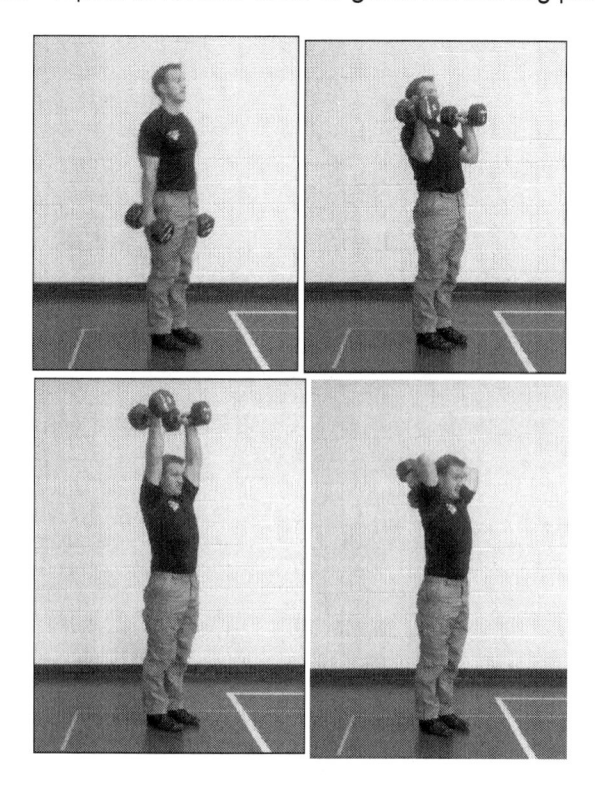

MJDB #2: Same as above but add in a squat when your hands are in the down bicep position (by your hips)

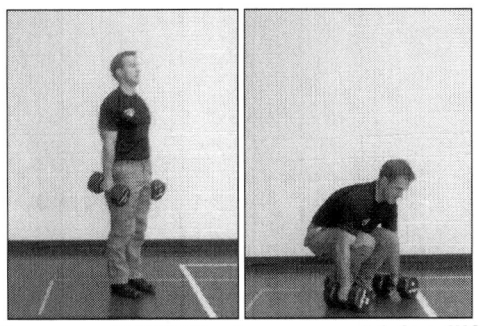

Same as MJDB#1 plus a squat / deadlift

MJDB #3: Same as MJDB #2 plus you add in a squat thrust and 1-5 push-ups. Five push-ups is recommended per cycle.

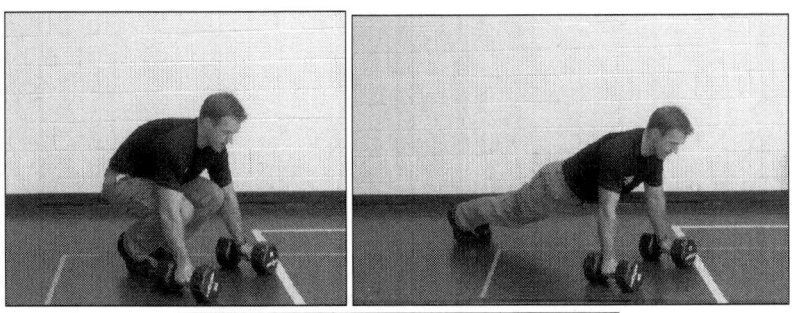

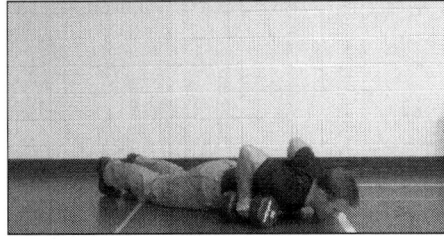

Repeat in reverse order and continue MJDB#2

Dead Lift / Power Clean Starting Position - Side View - Keep your head up, back straight, and lift with your legs, not only your back.

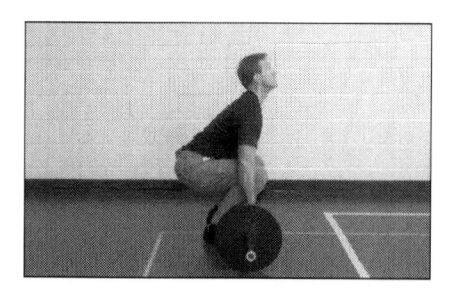

Dead Lift – With the barbell on the ground, place feet about shoulder width apart and bend down to grab the bar as shown. Keep your back straight and your head upright. Pull the barbell to your hips by standing (straighten legs and keep hips forward). Use the legs and hips to lift the weight NOT YOUR lower back. **DO NOT DO THIS EXERCISE WITH HEAVY WEIGHT IF YOU HAVE NEVER TRIED THIS EXERCISE. Try the MJDBs instead.**

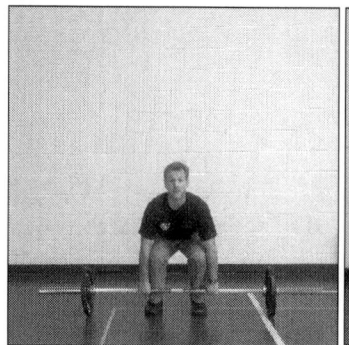

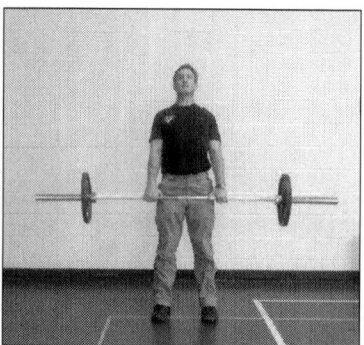

Power Clean is one of the most dynamic exercises in athletics. Make this movement fast and get the momentum of the barbell moving fast from the start so it is an easy transition with the power relay into the torso / arms.

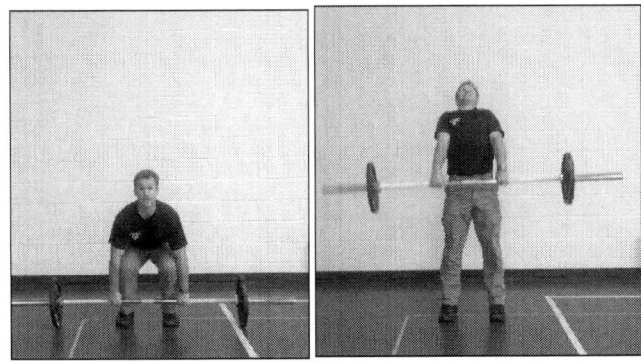

After you lift the bar off the ground, quickly get under the bar by squatting and racking the bar across your shoulders – then stand as in a ***front squat*** motion.

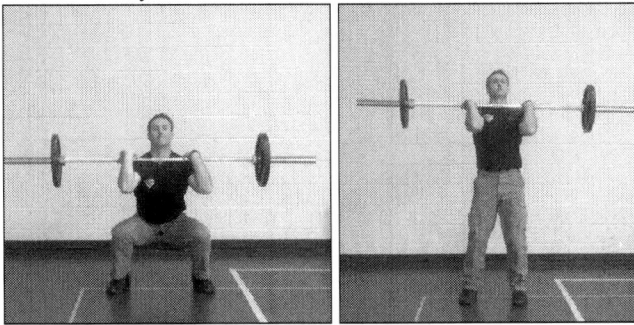

Hang clean - Pull the barbell to your hips by standing (straighten legs and keep hips forward – dead lift). Use the legs and hips to lift the weight NOT YOUR lower back. Now swing the barbell to the chest by bending your knees and dropping your waist 6-12 inches. Drop weight to your waist and repeat - DO WITH LIGHT WEIGHT BARBELL OR DUMBBELLS. (MJDBs for beginners to barbell lifting)

Hang Clean with Front Squat Option - as with the power clean the front squat is optional but a great addition to all muscle groups. With the bar stopped at your waist. Slowly drop a few inches and explode as you would do with a power clean. Hang clean is a power clean that starts with the barbell at your waist.

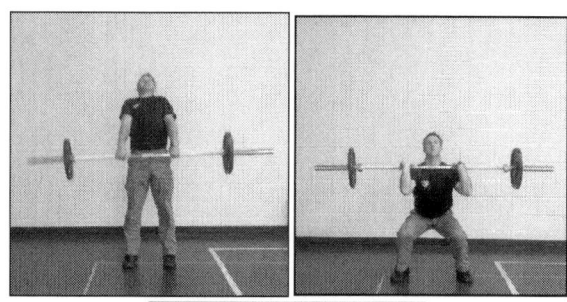

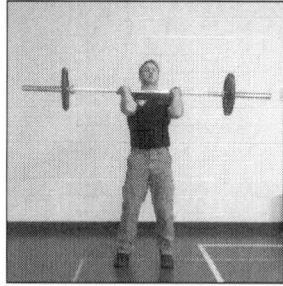

Log PT Simulation – You can replace the barbells if you have a log and do **push presses, dead lifts, and even hang cleans** with a log. Or to prepare for log PT, grab a barbell, dumbbell, and get good at overhead pushes, holds, and lifts off the ground. Remember – TEAMWORK!

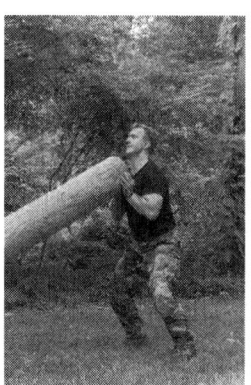

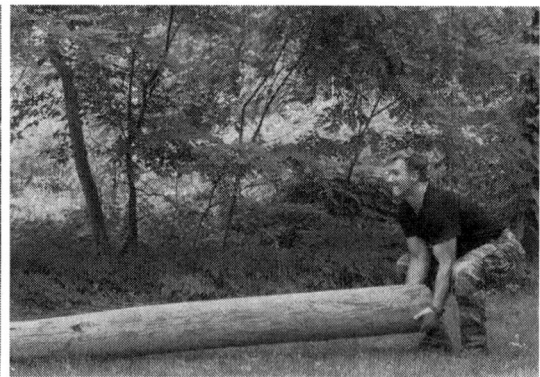

Fireman Carry Drills – Whether it is an injured man drill or a one on one fireman carry, learn to get good at placing a person on your shoulders and carrying him. This is a fun addition to the Burpee / 8 Count Pyramids with runs in between pullup bars. Instead of running every set, mix in some bear crawls and some fireman carries.

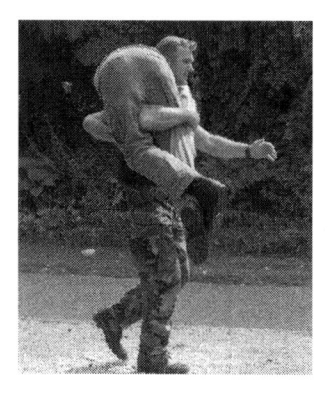

Thruster (front squat into over head press) – Explode upward from the front squat position straight into an overhead press or push press.

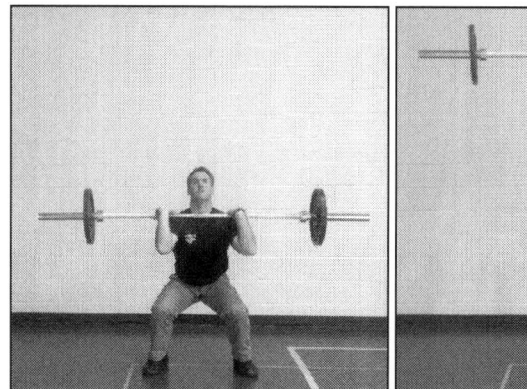

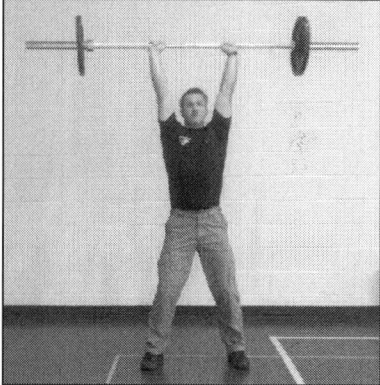

* The thruster is a deeper version of the "Push Press" exercise. You can opt to do the Push Press if you burn out with doing full squats but still have upper body left in the set.

Thrusters with dumbbells – You can do these with dumbbells as well or even a single plate. The goal is to squat and forcefully stand and use the momentum of the upward movement to easily lift the weight over your head

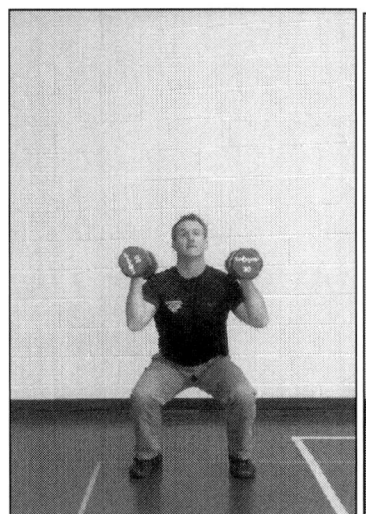

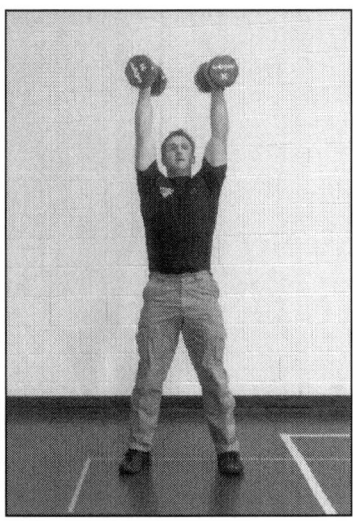

Farmer Walk – Grab a weight or sandbag with a handle in one hand and walk 100m changing hands at the 50m mark. This is great for grip as well as core strength.

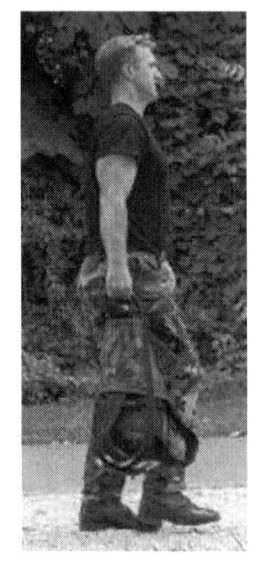

Chapter Seven: The Light Weight Shoulder Workout

This shoulder routine is great for post rotator cuff / shoulder surgery physical therapy patients. See link to video that explains all of the exercises in actual progression.

LATERAL RAISE: More than 5 pound dumbbells is not recommended for this exercise. Keep your shoulders back and your chest high. Lift weights parallel to ground in a smooth controlled motion, keep your palms facing the ground. Follow the next 6 exercises without stopping.

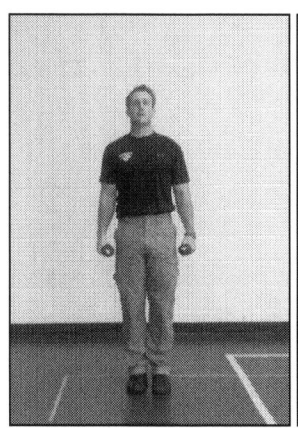

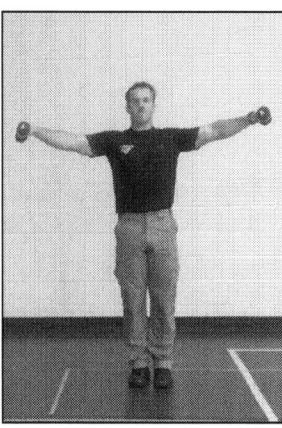

THUMBS UP: After performing 10 regular lateral raises, do 10 lateral raises with your thumbs up, touching your hips with your palms facing away from you and raising your arms no higher than shoulder height.

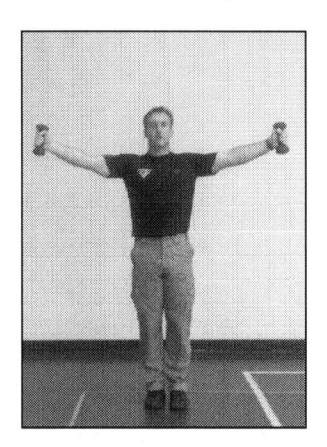

THUMBS-UP/DOWN: Continue with side lateral raises. As you lift your arms upward, keep your thumbs up. Once your arms are shoulder height, turn your hands and make your thumbs point toward the floor. Repeat for 10 times, always leading in the up and down direction with your thumbs.

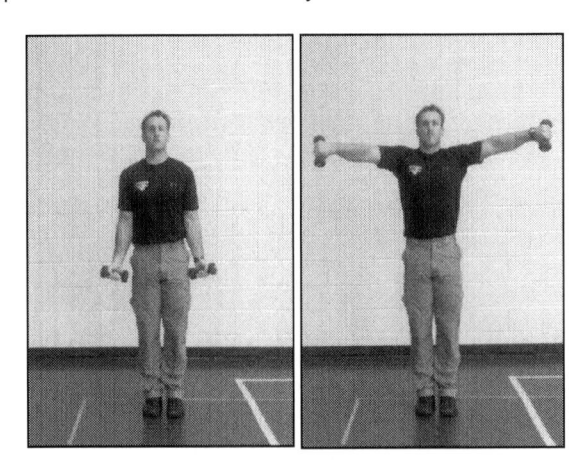

FRONT RAISE - THUMBS-UP: Now, for 10 more repetitions, to work your front deltoids. Lift the dumbbells from your waist to shoulder height keeping your thumbs up and arms straight.

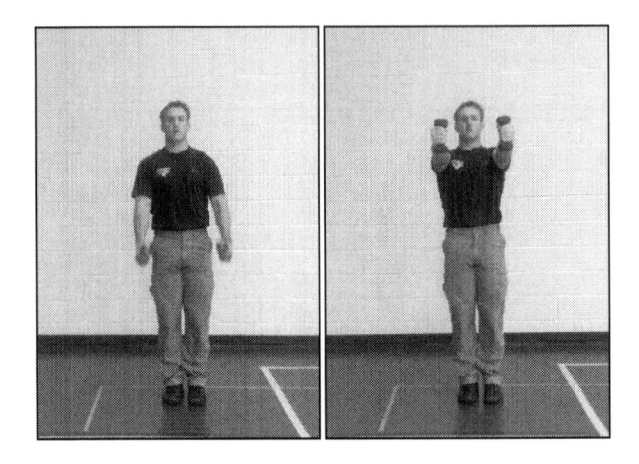

CROSS-OVERS: With your palms facing away from you and arms relaxed in front of your hips, bring your arms up and over your head as if you were doing a jumping jack (without jumping). Cross your arms IN FRONT of your head and bring them back to your hips for 10 repetitions.

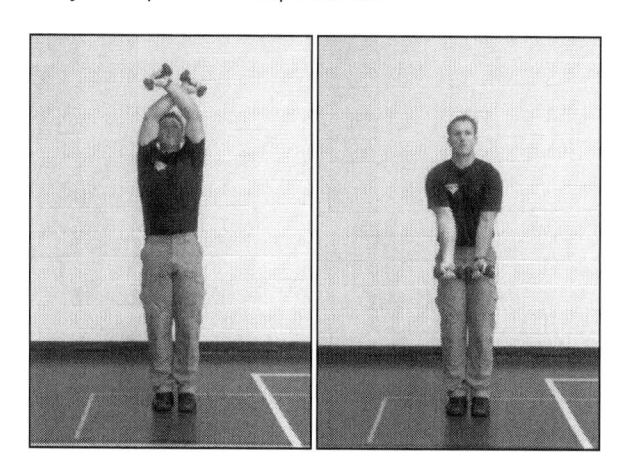

MILITARY PRESS: Place one foot ahead of the other as shown and knees slightly bent to reduce strain on your lower back. Exhale as you push the weights over your head for 10 final repetitions in the mega-shoulder pump workout. Slowly lower them to shoulder height and repeat. Muscles used are shoulders and triceps (back of arm).

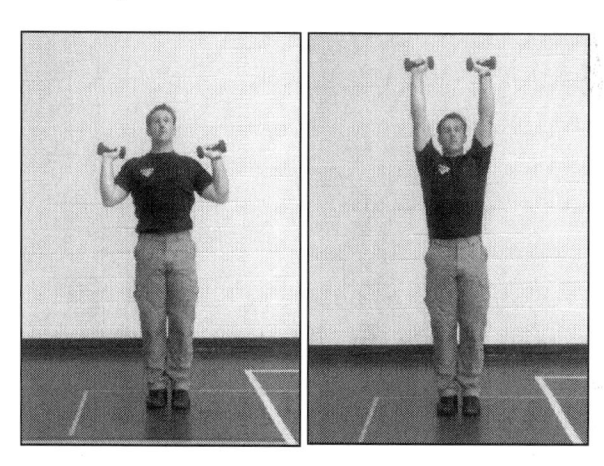

Section Three: Workouts and Explanations

This section is to help explain some of the workout designs. The goal in these workouts is to do what you can or have time for. If you do not a pool try another form of non-impact cardio options. If you have a pool but do not swim, try swimming some, but focus on the treading and dynamic stretching in the pool as this is exceptional for your hips, legs, and lower back. You can also work your shoulders and elbows as well by doing jumping jacks or other angled movements with your arms to work your joints in a full range of motion.

Chapter Eight: About The Workouts Specifics

Rest Day / Stretch
These are days to relax and stretch. Your body needs rest from rigorous exercise. In fact, it is the only way you will grow and get stronger. You should exercise 5 to 6 times per week and rest 1- 2 days per week. Skip a day if you feel the need or lack the time to complete all the workouts.

The Pyramid Workouts:

If you take a look at one of the pyramids, you will notice that it is numbered on both sides. It goes from 1-5 on one side, with the number 10 on the top, and then 9-1 on the other side. Each number represents a step in the pyramid. Your goal is to climb the pyramid all the way up, and all the way back down. So you can consider each step a "set" of your workout.

At the bottom, you will find "pullups x 1, pushups x 2, situps x 3". What this means is that at each "set" or step of the pyramid, you perform 1 pullup for every step you are on, 2 pushups for each step, and 3 situps for each step.

You start at the bottom of the pyramid, at number one. For each set, you times that set number by 1 and that tells you how many pullups to do. You multiply it by 2 to get your pushups, and multiply by 3 for situps. So you keep progressing until you get to the top of the pyramid, or your MAX At step ten you perform 10 pullups/ 20 pushups/30 situps. Now you start working your way back down the other side. So the next set you do will be at step 9 on the way back down. So, you'll do 9 pullups/18 pushups/27 situps. Keep going until you worked all the way back down to one. So here is a number summary of the pyramid:

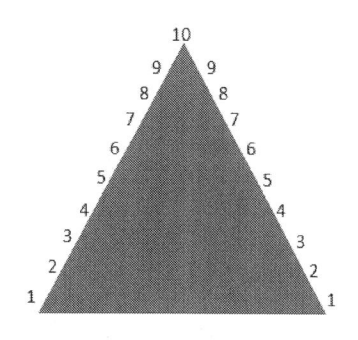

Go up the pyramid: (or half pyramid workout)
Set/Step 1: 1 pullups/2 pushups/3 situps
Set/Step 2: 2 pullups/4 pushups/6 situps
Set/Step 3: 3 pullups/6 pushups/9 situps
Set/Step 4: 4 pullups/8 pushups/12 situps
Set/Step 5: 5 pullups/10 pushups/15 situps   (Your first 5 sets are basically a warmup)
Set/Step 6: 6 pullups/12 pushups/18 situps
Set/Step 7: 7 pullups/14 pushups/21 situps
Set/Step 8: 8 pullups/16 pushups/24 situps
Set/Step 9: 9 pullups/18 pushups/27 situps
Set/Step 10: 10 pullups/20 pushups/30 situps

Once you have reached the top of the pyramid or failed at earlier levels, go down the pyramid: (repeat in reverse order pyramid = toughest to easiest number of reps)

The Pull-up Workouts:

The Pullup Pyramid: You will want to rest in between pull-up sets for no longer than one minute. Continue the pull-ups until you cannot perform any more - THEN resort to negatives for the remainder of the workout. In between sets, instead of resting and doing nothing, try to do at least 25 abdominal exercises of your choice or make it harder and do burpees or pushups in between sets of pullup pyramid sets.

100,200,300 PT Workout - The object of the 50 or 100 pullup, pushups, situps or squats workout is to do as many repetitions in as few sets as possible. Alternate exercises in a circuit fashion for quicker times to complete the workout. If you cannot do all the reps, you can also supplement rows, assisted pullups, or pulldowns in order to complete the 50-100 rep pullup workout if pure pullups at that volume are not possible – yet.

PT Pyramid Warmups – Find a place to do 15-25m of dynamic stretches in between exercises. Often burpee pyramid, squat / pushup pyramids will make up the warmup pyramid. Do 1 rep of exercise – run 25m – do 2 reps, run 25m..usually the pyramid will only go up to 5 or 10 sets. You do not have to repeat in reverse order down the pyramid unless it states.

10,20,30…Warmups – These are similar to the above pyramid warmup – just harder. Do 10 pushups and/or squats – run 200m (mix in some dynamic stretches) then to 20 pushups and/or squats – run 200m…keep going up 30,40, even 50 some days.

You can build up your strength and within a few months of this workout, you will have your first pullup in years - maybe ever!! Most people have a goal of achieving a pullup when they start working out again with this type of program.

You will see there are several different grips to use while doing pullups. This is to equally exercise every angle of the back, arms and forearms.

Circuit Workouts - You will see several different circuit routines in this workout program. Basically, a circuit workout is designed to move you as quickly through a workout as possible. There are no rest periods in a circuit until the end. Moving from one exercise to the other is the only rest you will get, but you will rarely be using the same muscle group two times in a row. So there is actually rest built into the workout.

8 Count body builder or Burpee / Pullup Pyramid – Obstacle Course prep workout without an obstacle course. Increase each set until you fail at pull-ups. Here is how the Pullup / 8 count body builder pyramid workout works:

Do ONE 8 count bodybuilder pushup (or burpee) - run 30m to a pullup bar - do 1 pullup. Run back to 8 count area and do TWO 8 counts - run back to pullup bar - do 2 pullups. Continue up the pyramid to 20 if you really want to challenge yourself. Another option is go to 10 and repeat in reverse order for time. We like to do this on a basketball court or a field with a pullup bar on it.

PT with the clock - This type of workout is designed to help students ace a physical fitness test of pullups, pushups, and sit-ups. By performing as many reps as you can of each exercise in a certain time limit, you will be learning the pace required to achieve 100 pushups and 100 sit-ups in two minutes. By using the clock as your training guide, you will become accustomed to doing maximum reps in a time period which will further increase your scores as you continue to practice this type of training.

Tabata Intervals – Do 20 second sprint / 10 second easy for timed sets in the workout – usually done on bike, elliptical, or rowing machines.

Life Cycle Workout – Riding a stationary bike with increasing resistance levels, place bike on manual mode. Start off at level 1 or 2 and increase the resistance every minute until failure. Then repeat in reverse order. If your bike increases up to 20 levels – increase resistance by 2 levels every minute. Otherwise, just increase by one level if bike tops out at 10-12 levels.

Chapter Nine: About Treading and Water Movements

If you have a pool…Consider Treading Water (video options)

Pool Mobility Day Off (full article)

Tread water for 10 minutes – Work on big scissor kicks, breast stroke kicks, and arm range of motion strokes (like jumping jacks off the bottom of the pool).

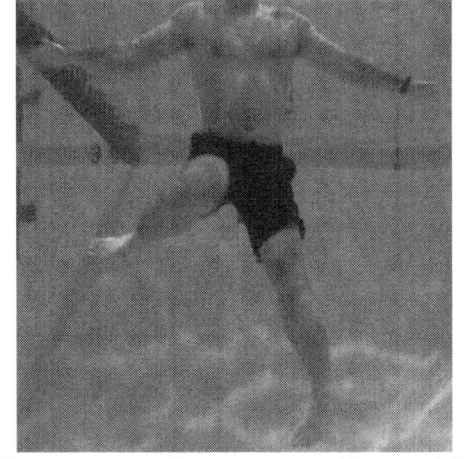

Then, like you do before you run with a warmup with a variety of dynamic stretches:

Try all dynamic stretches you do but in the pool in about chest-deep water (butt-kickers, Frankenstein walks, high knee lifts, leg swings (front / back / side to side).

Swim or tread water - 5 minutes

Butt Kickers - 1 minute

Frankenstein Walks - 1 minute

High Knee / Hip openers - 1 minute

Side Steps with hip opener – 1 min

Leg Swings Front / Back– 1 minute

Leg Swings (Left / Right) – 1 minute

(repeat with more options or longer time if needed)

DO NOT DO THESE WORKOUTS BY YOURSELF. IN FACT, NEVER SWIM UNDERWATER ALONE OR WITHOUT A LIFEGUARD.

Skip Breathing Swim pyramids (stroke per breath) This workout makes ordinary swimming seem easy and actually will help make swimming, running, and your overall endurance stronger.

This particular workout gets increasingly more difficult after each 100m you swim. By adding 2 strokes to your breathing pattern every 100m, you will find the need to breathe more demanding. Simply climb the pyramid making each set of 100m a step. Each step you will add two more strokes per breath. You will be breathing less per length on every step up the pyramid until you reach the maximum of 10 strokes per breath. A stroke is each arm pull, so the count would be this for a 4 strokes per breath step on the pyramid: 1,2,3,4, breathe - this translates to Left, right, left, right arm pull, breathe.

I find that if I hold my breath for at least half of the stroke count and then start exhaling slowly that I can make it through the pyramid with little difficulty. It does take time before you can do this workout with no rest at all. So, when you do this workout for the first few times, take about 20-30 seconds rest if you need to in between steps of the pyramid.

Swim Drills for Survival (drownproofing**)**

Tread water – using arms and legs relax and tread water. Try it without your hands, lifting your hands out of the pool for 5 minutes varying your kicks (flutterkicks, scissor kicks, breast stroke kicks, egg-beater kicks)

Bottom bounce – bounce off the bottom 20 times

Float – Keep hands and feet in same position and bend 90 degrees at the waist and float for 10-20 breaths.

Sequence of events for Swim Drills
treading – 5:00
floating – 5:00
bouncing 5:00

Swim PT - is a great way to squeeze in swimming and upper body PT into the same workout. Simply swim the specified distances (usually 100 yards or meters), get out of the pool and do pushups, abdominal exercises and pullouts. Repeat this sequence for at least 5-10 times.

Swim sprints

When the workout says sprints under swimming that means swim as fast as you can for the specified distance for the specified number of times. Try to limit your rest to no greater than 20-30 seconds. For instance: 200m x 3 means swim a 200m sprint, rest for 20-30 seconds and do it again two more times for a total of three times. Freestyle is the preferred stroke but you are free to choose the stroke you the wish to use. Swim Sprints with leg PT and upper body PT can also be incorporated into a hardcore swim/PT workout. If you mix leg PT with swimming try doing more flutter kicks and breast stroke kick swimming just to work the legs a little more as in the workout.

Run - Swim – Run or Ruck – The Spec Ops Triathlon

This one is as simple as the title on paper, but you will find the second run is a little more challenging, especially if you are swimming in fins. Try to do the run – swim –run in one workout period. It is not meant to be broken into 2 or 3 workouts. If that is your only way to do this workout then it is naturally OK to break up the workout to fit it in your schedule.

> 1) Run – 2 miles
> 2) Swim-2000m w/fins
> 3) Run 2 miles or Ruck 2 miles

Combat Swimmer Stroke (CSS) – OR MODIFIED SIDESTROKE

See video for moving version with FINS and without fins– **CSS link**

The CSS is a relaxing and efficient swim stroke that is an updated version of the traditional sidestroke. Whether you are a beginning swimmer or an aspiring Navy SEAL, this stroke can really help you efficiently move through the water.

The object to the CSS and side stroke is efficiency - you should try to get across a 25m pool in as few strokes as possible. If you are doing more than 10 strokes per length you are working too hard. In fact, the fastest and best swimmers get across a 25m pool in 3-5 strokes.

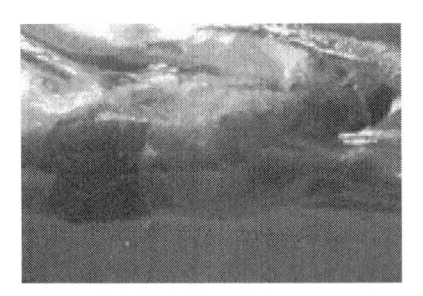

Side Stroke with Fins

Your hamstrings, hip flexors, and ankles will become strong after a few months of swimming with fins. It is similar to the side stroke without fins except you do **constant flutter-kicks** - With fins on your feet, your biggest source of power will naturally be your legs, so kick constantly in order to be propelled through the water. A picture is worth 1000 words, but when it comes to swimming, you need a video at least if you do not have an on-site coach.

An Efficient Video of the CSS – 1 minute.

Chapter Ten: The Workout Charts

The Program

This Tactical Fitness program will challenge you and may push you to failure many days. But, there are recovery days built into the middle of the week on Day 3 or Day 4. You still want workouts that will push your perceived limits, but you need at least one day off per week (5-6 workouts / week) and one of those days can be a Recovery Day. This is challenging, but not impossible. I promise you that you will be amazed at what you can do after you complete this sixteen week course. Do the stretches, foam rolling, dynamic warmups and water time for best results.

Running Supplement - Adding More To This Plan?

For those who are hardcore and need more mileage than in this program, add more miles on run and swim days or increase the workout with additional sets, reps if needed. Some ideas -
http://site.stewsmithptclub.com/6weekrunningplan.pdf

Running Replacement

Some people need LESS running mileage when starting a workout plan. If you are finding the running / speed workouts to be too much replace some of the runs with equal timed non-impact cardio events such as bike pyramid, elliptical and rowing tabata intervals, and swimming using the Running Non-Impact Replacement.

Good luck with the program and remember to consult your physician first before starting any program if you have not exercised in several months or years. If you need help with any fitness related questions please feel free to email me at stew@stewsmith.com.

The Workouts

The charts below contain sixteen weeks of workouts (4 x 4 different cycles) to help you prepare for the tactical life after 40. These can be done at any time of the year, we just tend to do this type of cycle in the corresponding seasons of the year:

Spring Cycle: Weeks 1-4: Calisthenics / Weight Training Mix and Running Progressions

Summer Cycle: Weeks 5-8: Calisthenics and Running Peak Progressions

Fall Cycle: Weeks 9-12: Transition into Weights / Reduce Calisthenics and Running

Winter Cycle: Weeks 13-16: Weight Training and Non-Impact Cardio Progression

Enjoy the workout charts below. They will challenge you and help you perform like you did decades before:

Weeks 1-4: Calisthenics / Weight Training Mix and Running

Spring - Week 1 – Calisthenics / Weights Mix – Running Build Up		
Day 1	Day 2	Day 3
Pushups / Squat Pyramid by 10s 10 pushups/10squats - run 200m, 20/20 pushups/squats run 200m, 30/30 pushups/squats run 200m...up to 50/50 **Repeat 5 times** Pullups max DB rows 10 Bench Press 10 Push press 10 DB Squats 10 DB lunges 10 Plank pose 1 min Light weight shoulders Run 1 mile Swimming Workout (optional – or bike 20 minute) 500m warmup swim (any stroke) **repeat 5 times** 100m sprint 1 min tread water 5 min dynamic stretches in chest deep water	Warmup 10 minutes bike / elliptical Stretch / Foam roll **Repeat 5 times** 5 min run or bike or elliptical or row 5 min stretch and foam roll Swim 15 minutes for max distance -_____ Tread water 5 minutes Do dynamic stretches in pool – chest deep water 5 minutes. (butt kickers, leg swings, Frankenstein kicks, etc..)	**Pushups / Squat Pyramid:** 10 pushups/10squats - run 200m, 20/20 pushups/squats run 200m, 30/30 pushups/squats run 200m...up to 50/50 5 min cardio warmup 2 min pullups* 2 min pushups* 2 min situps* 2 min burpees* 2 min squats* 2 min flutterkicks* 2 min walking lunges* 5 min cardio cooldown ***rest as needed but rest time counts = goal is to get as many reps of the exercises as you can in 2 minutes – exercises can be weighted too.** Run 1.5 mile Non-impact cardio of your choice 15 minutes / stretch

Week 1 - Calisthenics / Weights Mix – Running Build Up		
Day 4	Day 5	Day 6
Warmup 10 minutes bike / elliptical Stretch / Foam roll **Repeat 5 times** 5 min run or bike or elliptical or row 5 min stretch and foam roll **Repeat 2 times** Rev pushups - 20 Arm haulers - 20 Birds - 20 Swimmers - 30 secs Plank pose 1 min Swim 15 minutes for max distance -_____ Tread water 5 minutes Do dynamic stretches in pool – chest deep water 5 minutes. (butt kickers, leg swings, Frankenstein kicks, etc..)	Day off Pre-Test Taper Stretch	PFT Plus Warmup 10 min Pushups 1 min Situps 1 min Pullups max reps 1 mile run – timed 10 min break Bench Press – 5RM (max weight for 5 reps) Squats – 5RM (max weight 5 reps) DB Thrusters max reps 1 minute Cooldown 5 minute bike – top off with Reset PT **Repeat 2 times** Rev pushups - 20 Arm haulers - 20 Birds - 20 Swimmers - 30 secs Plank pose 1 min Stretch / Foam Roll this weekend

Week 2 - Calisthenics / Weights Mix – Running Build Up

Day 1	Day 2	Day 3
Pushups / Squat Pyramid: Run 200m, 10 pushup, 10 squat run 200m, 20 pushup/20 squats run 200m...up to 50 / 50. (by 10) Max Pullups Max Situps 2 min Light weight shoulders **Repeat 3 times** Bench Press 5-10 Pullups max DB rows 10/arm DB Thrusters 10 Plank pose 1 min DB Push press 10 Situps 1 min **Repeat 2 times** Rev pushups - 20 Arm haulers - 20 Birds - 20 Swimmers - 30 secs Plank pose 1 min Run 2 miles	Warmup 10 minutes bike / elliptical Stretch / Foam roll **repeat 5 times** 5 Min cardio - 5 min stretch or foam roll (mix in bike, elliptical, row, etc) Stretch / Foam roll	**Pushups / Squat Pyramid:** Run 200m, 10 pushup, 10 squat run 200m, 20 pushup/20 squats run 200m...up to 50 / 50. (by 10) Max Pullups Max Situps 2 min Light weight shoulders **Repeat 3 times** Pullups max DB rows 10/arm Dead lifts 5 **Repeat 3 times** Squats 10 Farmer walks up / down stairs 3x DB Thrusters 10 Flutterkicks 30 **Repeat 2 times** Rev pushups - 20 Arm haulers - 20 Birds - 20 Swimmers - 30 secs Plank pose 1 min Run 2 miles

Week 2 - Calisthenics / Weights Mix – Running Build Up		
Day 4	Day 5	Day 6
Warmup 10 minutes bike / elliptical Stretch / Foam roll **repeat 5 times** 5 Min cardio or choice 5 min stretch or foam roll (mix in bike, elliptical, row, etc) Stretch / Foam roll OR Cardio Option: run, bike, elliptical, rower, swim…30 minutes If swim – mix in 5 minute tread 5 minutes of dynamic stretches in chest deep water Stretch / Foam roll	**Pushups / Squat Pyramid**: Run 200m, 10 pushup /10 squat - run 200m, 20 pushup /20 squats - run 200m… up to 50 / 50. (by 10) Light weight shoulders **Upper Body Pyramid Plus** Pullups 2,4,6,8,10… Pushups 5,10,15,20,25 Sit-ups 5,10,15,20,25 Dips 2,4,6,8,10… *mix in bench press, plank poses (1 sec / rep) on some situps sets. Supplement pullups with DB rows or Pulldowns when needed to complete a failed set.* Keep going up until you fail at TWO exercises - then repeat in reverse order IF below 16 on pullups / dips - otherwise keep going up. **Run 2 miles**	**Big Cardio** Run 2 miles Ruck 2 miles Plus non- impact options 30 minutes swim, bike or elliptical tabata interval or pyramid workout If swim – tread water 5 minutes and dynamic stretches 10 minutes in chest deep water

Week 3 - Calisthenics / Weights Mix – Running Build Up

Day 1	Day 2	Day 3
Pushups / Squat Pyramid: Run 25m, 1 pushup/1 squat - run 25m, 2 pushup/2 squats - run 25...up to 5/5 – Warmup Light weight shoulders **Repeat 3 times** Pullups max Military press 10 **Repeat 3 times** bench press 10 dips max **Repeat 3 times** Squats 10 Wall sits 1 min **Repeat 3 times** Dead lift 5 Rows 10/arm MJDB#2-10 Run 2.5 miles **Or Swim** 500m warmup **Repeat 5 times** Swim 50m fast free Swim 50m CSS to catch breath - no rest Dynamic stretches 5 minutes in chest deep water	**Big Cardio** Run 2 miles or Ruck 2 miles Plus non-impact options Swim 1000m with fins OR 30 minutes bike or elliptical tabata intervals OR Row 3 x 5000m timed events - rest as needed **Repeat 2 times** Rev pushups - 20 Arm haulers - 20 Birds - 20 Swimmers - 30 secs Plank pose 1 min	**Fast Intervals / PT** Light weight shoulders **Repeat 5 times** 2 min sprint - run, bike, elliptical - fast as you can handle **THEN** (1 min on every exercise below in circuit: - 1 min: Pullups or pulldowns - 1 min: Pushups or dips, - 1 min: CHOICE: burpees, hang clean, power clean, KB swings, MJDB#2 or #3, - 1 min: Squats or lunges - 1 min: Abs of choice - Situps, flutterkicks leg levers, crunches, or plank pose Run 2 miles or bike 15 minutes Swim 500m **Repeat 5 times** 100m FAST - rest with 1 min tread Dynamic stretches 5 minutes in chest deep water

Week 3 - Calisthenics / Weights Mix – Running Build Up		
Day 4	Day 5	Day 6
Warmup 10 minutes bike / elliptical Stretch / Foam roll 10 min run 5 min stretch / foam roll 10 min bike or row / 5 min stretch / foam roll 10 min elliptical or run – 5 min stretch / foam roll 10 min tread - no hands Swim with fins 1000m **Repeat 2 times** Rev pushups - 20 Arm haulers - 20 Birds - 20 Swimmers - 30 secs Plank pose 1 min	Pushup/Squat Reverse pyramid 1-10: Pushups 1 / squats 1 – run 25m, Pushups 2 / squats 2 – run 25m..up to 10 <u>Light weight shoulders</u> **Repeat 3 times** Run 5 minutes Squats 20 Pullups max Pulldowns 10 Dips max Plank pose 1 min Bench Press 10 Rows 10/arm Flutterkicks 50 BIKE or elliptical 15-20 minutes SWIM **Repeat 5 times** Swim 100m timed - rest with abs of choice: 50 reps flutterkicks, leg levers, situps, crunches, etc... Tread 5 minutes Dynamic Stretches 10 minutes	Warmup 10 minutes bike / elliptical Stretch / Foam roll **Repeat 5 times** 5 min run or bike or elliptical or row 5 min stretch and foam roll Swim 15 minutes for max distance -_____ Tread water 5 minutes Do dynamic stretches in pool – chest deep water 5 minutes. (butt kickers, leg swings, Frankenstein kicks, etc..) **Repeat 2 times** Rev pushups - 20 Arm haulers - 20 Birds - 20 Swimmers - 30 secs Plank pose 1 min

Week 4 - Calisthenics / Weights Mix – Running Build Up		
Day 1	Day 2	Day 3
Warmup with 5 min cardio of your choice THEN **Repeat 5 times** Jumping jacks 10 Pushups 5-10 Squats 10 5 min cardio **Lift / PT Circuit:** **Repeat 2 times** Bench Press 10 Pullups 5-10 (or max) DB rows 10/arm 5 min cardio **Repeat 2 times** Pushups max Crunches 20 Military press 5-10 Pulldowns 10 5 min cardio **Repeat 2 times** Db thrusters 10 reps DB Lunges 5/leg MJDB#2 - 5-10 reps Cooldown 10-15 min non-impact cardio options: Bike, elliptical, row, or swim If Swim - tread 5 minutes and dynamic stretches in pool 5 min	**Cardio only Workout** - Do as many options below as you can Run 20 minutes and / or **Bike pyramid** - increase levels of resistance by 2 until failure to maintain 80 rpm on stationary bike - then return in reverse order to where you started **Elliptical** – how quickly can you burn 100 calories? ____ **Tabata intervals of 5-10 minutes of all the above options if available: (tabata = 20 sec sprint / 10 sec easy)** **Repeat 2 times** Rev pushups - 20 Arm haulers - 20 Birds - 20 Swimmers - 30 secs Plank pose 1 min	Warmup with 5 min easy cardio / light stretch **Fullbody Fitness Test:** **2 minute challenge:** 2 min pushups / rest in plank when not doing pushups 2 min crunches 2 min squats (weight vest optional 25#) 2 min plank pose (pass/fail) 2 min Pullups (rest as needed) max reps in 2 min period 2 min step ups (onto bench or box) 2 min burpees Run 2 min – sprint – how far do you get? Cardio cool down - bike, swim, elliptical 15-20 min If Swim: Tread 5 minutes Dynamic Stretches 10 minutes

Week 4 - Calisthenics / Weights Mix – Running Build Up

Day 4	Day 5	Day 6
Cardio only Workout - Do as many options below as you can Run / walk mix if needed - try 100yd jog / 100yd walk for as long as you can stand it - then just walk or jog mix for extra 20 minutes Bike pyramid - increase levels of resistance by 2 until failure to maintain 80 rpm on stationary bike - then return in reverse order to where you started Elliptical - same pyramid as above **Tabata intervals of 5-10 minutes of all the above options if available: (tabata = 20 sec sprint / 10 sec easy)**	Day off or Easy Cardio Day 1 mile run 10 min bike 10 min elliptical 10 min easy swim Tread water 5 min Dynamic stretches 5 minutes Stretch	Build Your Own PFT **Upper PT:** Pushups 1-2 min Pullups – Max reps Dips Max reps (pick 2) **Core PT**: Sit-ups 2 min Crunches 2 min Plank pose 2 min (p/f) (pick 1) **Upper Weights** BW Bench max reps 20# pullup max reps (pick 1) **Full body PT / WT** Burpee max - 2 min *KB swings - 5 min *Thrusters - 2 min (*50-75# weight) (pick 1) **Cardio**: 1.5 mile run 500m swim – any stroke 4 Mile Ruck 50# (pick 1 or 2) BW = bodyweight **PT Reset** **Repeat 2 times** Rev pushups - 20 Arm haulers - 20 Birds - 20 Swimmers - 30 secs Plank pose 1 min

Weeks 5-8: Calisthenics and Running Peak Progressions

Summer Cycle - Week 1 – Calisthenics / Running Phase		
Day 1	Day 2	Day 3
PT Pyramid: First 5 sets (1,2,3,4,5) mix in short runs of butt kicks, other dynamic stretches for 25yds. PT Pyramid: Pullups x 1, Pushups x 2, Abs of choice x 3 – 1-10-1 Light weight shoulders 2-3 mile timed run Or Non-impact 20 min bike, elliptical, rower or Swim Workout 500m warmup **Repeat 5 times** 100m sprint free 50m CSS or breaststroke - easy	Non-impact option today if available: **Repeat 5 times** Bike or elliptical 5 min fast tabata interval - Air Squats 20 - Air Lunges 10/leg Or run ½ mile in place of tabata interval if you prefer to run and do leg PT/lift Ruck 2 mile or swim with fins 1000m to top off leg day Do dynamic stretches in pool – chest deep water 5 minutes. (butt kickers, leg swings, Frankenstein kicks, etc..)	Warmup with short run 1 mile **Repeat 10 times** Jumping jacks 10 Pushups 10 PT Super Set: **Repeat 5-10 times** Run ¼ mile or 2 min bike / elliptical.. Pullups 5-10 Pushups 10-20 Situps 10-20 Dips 10 Plank pose 1 min Light weight shoulders **Repeat 2 times** Rev pushups - 20 Arm haulers - 20 Birds - 20 Swimmers - 30 secs Swim 500m timed any stroke - tread water – no hands 5 minutes Swim 500m timed again

Week 1 - Calisthenics Phase		
Day 4	Day 5	Day 6
Warmup bike or job 5 minutes / stretch **Repeat 5 times** Run, Bike or elliptical 5 min fast tabata Foam roller 2 minute **Optional**: Ruck with 30-40# - fast walk/shuffle – steady pace – 30 minutes OR Swim 1000m with fins – any stroke *If pool available* – tread water 10 minutes – then doing all dynamic stretches in the pool you normally do on land	Warmup with 1.5 mile run **/ stretch when needed.** **Max Rep PT:** First 5 sets mix in short runs of butt kicks, other dynamic stretches for 25yds. (keep track of reps 1,2,3,4,5 = 15 reps) Pullups 100 Pushups 200 Abs of Choice 300 Dips 200 Run 1.5 miles Light weight shoulders *add in some TRX pushups / TRX rollouts for abs options / TRX rows if needed for pullups.	Make up day or run / ruck and/or swim event of your choice of distance / time. **Spec Ops Tri** Run 1 miles or elliptical 10 minutes Ruck 1 miles or bike 10 minutes Swim 1000m with fins. **Repeat 2 times** Rev pushups - 20 Arm haulers - 20 Birds - 20 Swimmers - 30 secs Plank pose 1 min

Week 2 - Calisthenics Phase

Day 1	Day 2	Day 3
Warmup with pullup x1 / pushups x2 / situps x 3 pyramid to 5 levels (dynamic stretches after each set for 25m) Max Pullups Max Pushups - 2 min Max Situps 2 min Run 1 mile or bike 10 minutes Max Pullups Max Pushups until you have to rest - stay in plank for extra 1 min Max Situps 1 min Run 1 mile or row 10 minutes Max Pullups Max Pushups until you have to rest - stay in plank for extra 1 min Max Situps 1 min Run 1 mile or elliptical 10 minutes **Repeat 2 times** Rev pushups - 20 Arm haulers - 20 Birds - 20 Swimmers - 30 secs Plank pose 1 min	**Run and Leg PT:** **Repeat 5 times** Squats – 10 then short runs of butt kicks, other dynamic stretches for 25yds. Run or bike 15 minutes -how far do you get? **Repeat 5 times** run 200m fast squats 20 **Repeat 5 times** run 400m fast lunges 10/leg 5-10 minutes of bike or elliptical cooldown Or swim 500m-1000m with fins Tread water 5 min Dynamic stretches 5 minutes in chest deep water.	Warmup 5 min jog Pullups, 2,4,6,8,10 - do 10 pushups / 10 situps in between pullups **Repeat 2 times** pushups 1 min situps 1 min pullups max dips max run 1 mile or bike 10 minutes **Repeat 2 times** Pushups Situps 1 min Pullups max Dips max 100-200m sprint Light weight shoulders **Repeat 2 times** Rev pushups - 20 Arm haulers - 20 Birds - 20 Swimmers - 30 secs 100-200m sprint **Swim Cooldown Option** Swim 500m Plank pose 1 min Flutterkicks 1 min Swim 500m with fins

Week 2 - Calisthenics Phase		
Day 4	Day 5	Day 6
Mobility / Recovery Warmup 5 minute easy bike or elliptical 10 min bike 10 min elliptical 10 min row or 10 min tread in pool (5 min all arms / 5 min all leg tread) If pool: Swim 500m without fins Do dynamic stretches in pool – chest deep water 5 minutes. (butt kickers, leg swings, Frankenstein kicks, etc..)	**Run and PT Mix (Push / Pull / Sprint)** **Repeat 5 times** Pullups max effort Pushups – max effort for 1 minute 50m easy jog 100m sprint 50m easy jog 100m sprint Abs of choice 2 min Light weight shoulders **Repeat 2 times** Rev pushups - 20 Arm haulers - 20 Birds - 20 Swimmers - 30 secs Swim or Other Cardio **Swim Cooldown Option** Swim 500m Pushups 1 min Plank pose 1 min Flutterkicks 1 min Swim 500m with fins *If other cardio, run, bike, elliptical, or row tabata interval for 5 minutes – three times.	**Run and Leg and Swim PT** Run 1/4 mile warmup / stretch (dynamic stretches after each set for 25m) Lunges 10 / leg Run 1/2 mile stretch Lunges 10/legs Run 3/4 mile stretch Lunges 10/leg Run 1/2 mile timed stretch Run 1/4 mile at goal mile pace **Swim Workout:** **Repeat 5 times** 100yds at 6-8 strokes per breath freestyle squats 20 Tread water 5 min Do dynamic stretches in pool – chest deep water 5 minutes. (butt kickers, leg swings, Frankenstein kicks, etc..)

Week 3 - Calisthenics Phase		
Day 1	Day 2	Day 3
PT Max Reps Set with Runs **Warmup with 1-10 burpee pyramid** / stretch - run 25m in between each set doing dynamic stretches Light weight shoulders **Repeat 5-10 times** Pullups 10 Pushups 20 Abs of choice max in 1 minute (TRX or other) Run 400m fast **Repeat 2 times** Rev pushups - 20 Arm haulers - 20 Birds - 20 Swimmers - 30 secs 2 mile easy pace cooldown run or 20 minute swim / bike or elliptical If you swim: Do 5 min tread and 5 minute dynamic stretches to end workout.	20 min easy bike or elliptical **Repeat 5 times** 3 min bike, row or elliptical 10 squats 10 lunges / leg **Cool down non-impact cardio 10 minutes** Dynamic stretches 5 minutes	PT Max Reps Sets with Crawls / Runs **Repeat 5-10 times** Pullups max Stair crawls up/down Pushups max *In other words:* *pullups - supplement with TRX rows if needed to get 15-20 reps each set* *staircrawls up/down or bear crawl 50m* *pushups how many reps can you get in as few sets as possible.* **Repeat 6 times** 400m fast 50 abs of choice or 1 min plank pose **Cool down non-impact cardio 10 minutes** Dynamic stretches 5 minutes Or Swim 500m fast tread water 5 minutes then dynamic stretches 5 minutes.

Week 3 - Calisthenics Phase		
Day 4 – Mobility Day	Day 5	Day 6
Dynamic Stretches 10 minutes (butt kickers, Frankenstein walks, side steps, high knees, bounding, etc) **Repeat 5 times** 5 min bike or elliptical steady pace 5 min foam roller and stretch combo Pool: 500m swim tread 5 minutes Dynamic stretches 10 minutes in chest deep water. If no pool – do dynamic and static stretches 10 minutes as a cooldown	Burpee Pyramid Warmup 1-5: 1 burpee, run 25m, 2 burpee, run 25m RUN = Dynamic Stretches for 25m of (butt kickers, Frankenstein walks, side steps, high knees, bounding, etc) Light weight shoulders **Repeat 3 times** Run 1 mile Max Pullups Max Pushups Max plank pose or abs of choice 1 min **Repeat 2 times** Rev pushups - 20 Arm haulers - 20 Birds - 20 Swimmers - 30 secs **Cool down non-impact cardio 10-15 minutes** **Stretch – Pool cooldown optional**	Day off or non impact day Take a mobility day off Stretch 10-15 min Roam Roll 10-15 min this weekend

Week 4 - Calisthenics Phase

Day 1	Day 2	Day 3
PT Pyramid with Runs Pullups x 1, Pushups x 2, Abs of choice x 3 (or do with TRX options **some** sets - not all) Pullups x 1 (or TRX Rows) Pushups x 2 (or TRX atomic pushups) Situps x 3 (or TRX Rollouts) But – every 5 sets – run 1 mile or bike / elliptical / row 7 min tabata interval Light weight shoulders **Repeat 2 times** Rev pushups - 20 Arm haulers - 20 Birds - 20 Swimmers - 30 secs Plank pose 1 min **Pool: 500m swim** Tread 5 minutes no hands then Dynamic stretches 5 minutes in chest deep water. If no pool – do dynamic and static stretches 10 minutes as a cooldown	**Run / Squat pyramid:** 10 squats - run 200m*, 20 squats - run 200m, 30 squats - run 200m 40 squats - run 200m 50 squats - run 200m ***or bike 1 min fast*** Stretch **Repeat 5 times** Run or bike 3 min plank pose 1 min stretch 1 min 30 min run, swim with fins, bike, or elliptical If pool: Dynamic stretches 5 minutes in chest deep water.	**"Warmup" Pyramid** 10 pushups * 20 pushup * 30 pushups * - max Pullups 40 pushup * 50 pushup * - max Pullups * run 200m in btwn sets Light weight shoulders Run 1 mile Pushups max Situps max 1 min Pullups max Run 1 mile Pushups max Situps max 1 min Pullups max Run 1 mile Pushups max Plank pose 1 min Pullups max **Repeat 2 times** Rev pushups - 20 Arm haulers - 20 Birds - 20 Swimmers - 30 secs Plank pose 1 min **Pool: 500m swim** Tread 5 minutes no hands then Dynamic stretches 5 minutes in chest deep water.

Week 4		
Day 4	Day 5	Day 6
Easy Leg Day w/Mobility / Recovery 10 min bike or elliptical warmup **Repeat 3 times** Bike 3 minutes squats 20 **Repeat 3 times** Bike 3 minutes lunges 10/leg Pool or Dry Land Dynamic Stretches 10 minutes (butt kickers, Frankenstein walks, side steps, high knees, bounding, etc) Cooldown– easy cardio 10 minutes bike, elliptical, or swim (tread 5 min too) if you swim. Stretch	**"Warmup" Pyramid** 10 pushups * 20 pushup* 30 pushups* - max Pullups 40 pushup* 50 pushup * * run 200m in btwn sets Light weight shoulders Run 1 mile 100 pullups or DB rows Run 1 miles 100 pushups Run 1 mile 200 abs of choice or 5 minute plank pose spread throughout the workout above Stretch 5 min Foam roller legs 5 minutes	Warmup bike or job 5 minutes / stretch **Repeat 5 times** Run 5 min fast or Bike or elliptical 5 min fast tabata Foam roller 2 minute **Repeat 2 times** Rev pushups - 20 Arm haulers - 20 Birds - 20 Swimmers - 30 secs Plank pose 1 min **Optional**: Ruck with 30-40# - fast walk/shuffle – steady pace – as long as you prefer. OR Swim 1000m with fins – any stroke *If pool available* – tread water 10 minutes – then doing all dynamic stretches in the pool you normally do on land

Weeks 9-12: Transition into Weights / Reduce Calisthenics / Running

Fall - Week 1 – Calisthenics to Lifting Transition / Less Running		
Day 1	Day 2	Day 3
PT Super Sets with Runs **Warmup with 1-10 burpee pyramid** / stretch - run 25m in between each set doing dynamic stretches **Repeat 10 times** Pullups / Pulldowns 10 (mix in needed) Pushups / Bench Press 10-20 Abs of choice 30 or 30 sec plank pose Run 200m fast 2 mile easy pace cooldown run **Repeat 2 times** Rev pushups - 20 Arm haulers - 20 Birds - 20 Swimmers - 30 secs Plank pose 1 min **Swim PT workout:** **Repeat 5 times** Swim 150m fast pick one exercise to do 20 reps of (pushups, abs of choice or 1 min plank) -10 min tread no hands	2 mile easy run **Repeat 5 times** Run 200m fast squats 20 **Repeat 5 times** run 200m fast lunges 10/leg Swim 500m without fins timed **Swim Workout** **Swim with fins - 20 min** Tread water – no hands 5 minutes Dynamic stretches in pool – chest deep water 10 minutes	PT Super Set with Crawls / Runs **Repeat for 30 min** Bench Press 10 Situps or abs 30 Pullups 10 or Pulldowns 10-15 Stair crawl up/down flight of steps or bear crawl 25m Run 300m fast Easy run 2 miles **Repeat 2 times** Rev pushups - 20 Arm haulers - 20 Birds - 20 Swimmers - 30 secs Plank pose 1 min **Swim PT workout:** **Repeat 5 times** Swim 100 fast free at 8-10 strokes / breath Swim 50m CSS

Fall - Week 1 – Calisthenics to Lifting Transition / Less Running

Day 4	Day 5	Day 6 – Day off
1.5 mile easy run **Repeat 5 times** Run 400m squats 20 **Repeat 5 times** run 400m lunges 10/leg Dynamic Stretches 10 minutes (butt kickers, Frankenstein walks, side steps, high knees, bounding, etc) Swim 500m without fins timed **Swim Workout** **Swim with fins - 20 min** Tread water – no hands 5 minutes Dynamic stretches in pool – chest deep water 10 minutes	**Max Reps Sets** **Do 100,200,300 in as few sets as possible in circuit fashion.** Run 1 mile 100 pullups or pulldowns / rows when fail 200 pushups 300 abs of choice or 5 minute plank pose Run 1 mile Swim 500m warmup **Repeat 5 times** 200m sprint plank pose 1 min or 30 abs of choice	Day 7 **Double PST of your Choice (repeat in reverse order)** 500yd swim Pushups Situps Pullups 1.5 mile run **#2 options** Pushups Situps Pullups 1.5 mile run **#3 option:** Pushups Situps Pullups 2,3,4 or 5 mile run **#4 option:** 5 mile ruck or 1500m swim with fins or both

Fall - Week 2 – Calisthenics to Lifting Transition / Less Running

Day 1	Day 2	Day 3
Warmup with pyramid pushups / run sets: 1 pushups / 25m run, 2 pushups/25m run up to 20. - stop. **DB Circuit:** **Repeat 3 times** Cardio 5 minutes Pullups max Db rows 10 KB swings 20 MJDB#2 - 10 Plank pose 1 min (all non stop) **Weight Circuit:** **Repeat 4 times** Pullups max Pulldowns 10-15 Rows 10/arm Bench press 5-10 Pushups max Situps 1 min / goal pace Push press 10-15 Run 3 miles **Swim** 500m warmup **Repeat 10 times** Swim 75m fast free Swim 50m CSS to catch breath - no rest Tread 5 min Dynamic Stretches 5 min in water	Warmup with pyramid/run sets of squat / run pyramid: 1 squat - run 25m - 2 squats - run 25m...go up to 20 reps 30 min run 30 min Ruck Swim with fins 2000m	Warmup with 5 min cardio of choice Lightweight Shoulders **Weight Vest Wed:** Reverse Pyramid 20,19,18,17,16 - Pushups and plank pose / second with 25m run in between **15,14,13,12,11:** Dips, abs of choice, pushups - no run in between **10,9,8,7,6:** pullups, pushups, plank pose 1 min each set) **Drop weight vest:** 5,4,3,2,1: Bench press, heavy rows, pulldowns (Heavy) Run 3 miles And / or Swim 500m **Repeat 5 times** 250m FAST - rest with 1 min tread / float or bottom bounce. Tread 5 min Dynamic Stretches 5 min in water

Fall - Week 2 – Calisthenics to Lifting Transition / Less Running

Day 4	Day 5	Day 6
Warmup with pyramid/run sets of squat / run pyramid: 1 squat - run 25m - 2 squats - run 25m...go up to 20 reps 20 min bike or elliptical Swim with fins 1000m Tread water 10 minutes with fins Dynamic Stretches 5 minutes in pool	Warmup with pyramid pushups / run sets: 1 pushups / 25m run, 2 pushups/25m run up to 20. - stop. **Repeat 4 times** 5 minute cardio of choice Pushups 1 min Pullups max Bench press 5-10 Pulldowns 5-10 **Lightweight Shoulders** **Repeat 3 times** Military press 5-10 Situps 1 min Rows 5 / arm (heavy) Arm haulers 20 1 min overhead plate hold Plank pose 1 min **Swim PT** **Swim 500m warmup** **Repeat 5 times** Swim 100m timed - rest with abs of choice: 50 **reps flutterkicks, leg levers, situps, crunches, plank pose 1 min...**	Big Cardio Run 3 miles or Ruck 3 miles Plus non impact options Swim 1000m with fins Tread 5 min Dynamic Stretches 5 min in water OR 30 minutes bike or elliptical tabata interval OR Row 3 x 5000m timed events - rest as needed **Repeat 2 times** Rev pushups - 20 Arm haulers - 20 Birds - 20 Swimmers - 30 secs Plank pose 1 min

Fall - Week 3 – Calisthenics to Lifting Transition / Less Running

Day 1	Day 2	Day 3
Pushups / Squat Pyramid: Run 200m, 10 pushup, 10 squat run 200m, 20 pushup/20 squats run 200m...up to 50 / 50. (by 10) Max Pullups Max Situps 2 min **Repeat 5 times** Cardio of choice 5 minutes (run, bike, elliptical, row, steps, etc) Bench press 10 reps Pullups max Rows 10.arm Push press 10-15 Situps 1 min Run 3 miles **Swim** 500m warmup **Repeat 10 times** Swim 50m fast free Swim 100m CSS - rest with tread if needed	Warmup 10 minutes bike / elliptical Stretch / Foam roll **repeat 5 times** 5 Min cardio - 5 min stretch or foam roll (mix in bike, run, elliptical, row, etc) Swim with fins 1500m	**Pushups / Squat Pyramid:** Run 200m, 10 pushup, 10 squat run 200m, 20 pushup/20 squats run 200m...up to 50 / 50. (by 10) Max Pullups Max Situps 2 min **Repeat 3 times** Pullups max dead lifts 5 **Repeat 3 times** Farmer walks / stairs MJDB#2 - 15 **Repeat 3 times** Hanging Knee ups 20 Flutterkicks 50 ——— Run 3 miles Swim 500m **Repeat 7 times** 200m FAST - rest with 1 min tread / float or bottom bounce. 100m swim cooldown 5 min tread 5 min dynamic stretch in water

Fall - Week 3 – Calisthenics to Lifting Transition / Less Running		
Day 4	Day 5	Day 6
Warmup 10 minutes bike / elliptical Stretch / Foam roll **Repeat 4 times** 5 min run or bike or elliptical fast intervals 5 min stretch / foam roller 10 min tread - no hands Swim with fins 1500m	**Pushups / Squat Pyramid**: Run 200m, 10 pushup /10 squat - run 200m, 20 pushup /20 squats - run 200m... up to 50 / 50. (by 10) **Upper Body Pyramid Plus** Pullups 2,4,6,8,10... Pushups 5,10,15,20,25 Situps 5,10,15,20,25... Dips 2,4,6,8,10... Keep going up until you fail at TWO exercises - then repeat in reverse order IF below 16 on pullups / dips - otherwise keep going up. **SWIM** **500m warmup swim** **Repeat 5 times** Swim 250m timed - rest with abs of choice: 50 reps flutterkicks, leg levers, situps, crunches, etc...	**Big Cardio** Run 3 miles Ruck 3 miles Plus non impact options Swim 1500m with fins OR (in place of run or ruck) 30 minutes bike or elliptical tabata interval OR Row 3 x 5000m timed events - rest as needed

Fall - Week 4 – Calisthenics to Lifting Transition / Less Running

Day 1	Day 2	Day 3
Push, Pull, Leg, Full, Core/Grip, Cardio **1 min sets:** pushups 1 min Pullups 1 min Squats 1min Burpees 1min Situps 1 min Cardio 5 min **Repeat 3 times** bench press 1 min Pullups 1 min Squats, lunges or leg press 1 min MJDB#2 - 1 min or Thrusters 1 min Plank pose 1 min Cardio 5 min Lightweight Shoulder **Repeat 2 times** Rev pushups - 20 Arm haulers - 20 Birds - 20 Swimmers - 30 secs Plank pose 1 min Ruck or swim 30 minutes for max distance.	Bike / elliptical 20 minute warmup Run 20 minutes or bike/elliptical if you prefer Swim: 15 minute tread warmup - mix in dynamic stretches / exercises. 500m timed CSS or free How far can you swim with fins for 30 minutes? Lower back plan - do it later in the evening	Warmup 5 min **Push, Pull, Leg, Full, Core/Grip, Cardio** **Repeat 3 times** Bench press 5 Pullups 5-10 (wt) Squats - 5-10 Hang Clean 5-10 Plank 1 min Run or bike 5 min **Repeat 2 times** Rev pushups - 20 Arm haulers - 20 Birds - 20 Swimmers - 30 secs Plank pose 1 min Lightweight Shoulder Pullups - max swim 30 minutes for max distance.

Fall - Week 4 – Calisthenics to Lifting Transition / Less Running		
Day 4	Day 5	Day 6
Bike or Run 10-15 min warmup / stretch Make Up Day OR recovery day Non impact Cardio of your choice – bike, elliptical, row, swim for 20 minutes – pick 2 or 3 if you prefer to go an hour. *If pool option*– tread water 10 minutes – then doing all dynamic stretches in the pool you normally do on land	Sand Baby Murph PLUS **Repeat 5 times** Pullups max DB rows 10/arm Push Press 20 with 30-40# sandbag Lunges 10/leg Squats 20 Run 1/4 mile with sand baby on shoulder (30-40lbs sandbag) Bike or swim 30 minutes for max distance. If swim add in tread 10 minutes (5 min all arms / 5 min all legs) Dynamic Stretches 5 minutes in pool	Bike or Run 10-15 min warmup / stretch **Run - Ruck** 4 mile run and / or 4 mile ruck If available - find a hill and mix in a few hill run / rucks during the workout. Lower back plan - do it later in the evening

Weeks 13-16: Weight Training and Non-Impact Cardio Progression

Winter - Week 1 – Lifting / Non-Impact Cycle		
Day 1	Day 2	Day 3
Warmup with 10 min run or bike **5 x 5 Plus Pullups** Bench 5 x 5 *(Five sets of five reps) - 30 pullups - can be broken up during the 5 sets above. 5 min tabata intervals bike or elliptical Squats 5 x 5 - 30 pullups 5 min tabata interval bike or elliptical Dead Lifts 5 x 5 - 30 Pullups 5 min tabata interval bike or elliptical or row *do 30 pullups total during 5 x 5 sets Swim 100m warmup **Repeat 5-10 times** 50m sprint free 50m CSS @goal pace.	Cardio <u>20 min bike Pyramid</u> - each minute is tougher than previous minute. 20 min run or replace with 30 min ruck 5 min tread without hands 1000-1500m swim with fins **Upper Core Spread throughout workout:** **Repeat 3 times** - Rev. pushups 20 - Birds 20 - Arm Haulers - Plank Pose 1 min	Pushup / Squat pyramid 1-15 warmup - run 25m 1 pushup / 1 squat, run 25m 2 pushups, 2 squats...keep going to 15/15. Every 5th set do max pullups **LIFT:** **Repeat 3 times** Bench press 5 Pullups (weighted) 5 Hang Clean w/ Front Squat 5 Situp or plank pose - 1 min 20 min run or bike pyramid **Swim**: 5 min tread - no hands 5 min tread with fins - with weight (10-20lbs) Swim 500m with fins Swim 500m without fins for time. Dynamic Stretches in chest deep water 5 minutes

Winter - Week 1 – Lifting / Non-Impact Cycle		
Day 4	Day 5	Day 6
Core / Non-impact Cardio Day 20 min bike Pyramid - each minute is tougher than previous minute. **Repeat 3 times** 5 min tabata intervals on bike, elliptical or rower 5 min foam roller or stretch SWIM (optional) 5 minutes tread without hands 1000m swim with fins Dynamic Stretches in chest deep water 5 minutes As desired - throughout cardio events - stop and do a set of abs / plank pose.	Warmup with 10 min run or bike **Repeat 3 times** 5 min Tabata (bike or elliptical) Pullups (wt) max Bench press 5 Squats 5 or overhead lunges 10/leg Dead lift 5 Power Clean 5 Light stretch Cooldown 10 min run or bike **Swim**: 500m warmup **Repeat 5 times** 100m CSS @goal pace for 500m Pushups / Plank pose for the time it takes to swim 100m	**Run - Ruck Day** 2 mile run and / or 2 mile ruck If available - find a hill and mix in a few hill run / rucks during the workout. **Or Swim 1 hour** with fins and without fins / rest with skills like treading, dynamic stretches in water Lower back plan - do it later in the evening

Winter - Week 2 – Lifting / Non-Impact Cycle

Day 1	Day 2	Day 3
Push Pull Full Warmup with 1-10 Burpee Pyramid - run 25m in between. Lightweight Shoulder **Repeat 4 times** Pullups max Rows 10/arm Bench press 5-10 Pushups max Hang clean 5 Push press 10 Fireman carry 50m or farmer walk 100m Dips max Run 2 miles Swim 10 x 200m swims - rest with tread or bottom bounce 1 min in between	Leg Day Squat pyramid 1-10 - run 25m in btwn Squat pyramid 1-10 up/down flight of stairs: 1 squat - run up/down stairs, 2 squats up/down stairs...up to 10 - stop. Run or ruck 30 minutes THEN 1500m swim with fins. Can you get 2000m? Lower back plan - do it later in the evening	Warmup Burpee pyramid 1-10 dips 50 - rest with 50 abs when needed pullups 50 - rest with plank pose as needed Lightweight Shoulder **Repeat 3-4 times** Bench press 5-10 Pushups max Pullups max Pulldowns 10 Hang Clean 5 Push Press 10 Rows 10/arm Run 2 miles Swim 500m 5 min tread - no hands 1000m intervals of your choice.

Winter - Week 2 – Lifting / Non-Impact Cycle

Day 4	Day 5	Day 6
Run 30 minutes Swim up to 3000m with fins Break as as needed: 500m with fins / 500m without fins / work on free style, CSS, dolphin underwater kicks, etc.. Or take 10 minutes - tread with fins - holding 10lbs weight in place of 1 x 500m swim <u>Lower back plan - do it later in the evening</u>	**50 / 50 Full body** Warmup with 1-10 Burpee Pyramid with 25m run in between Continue - do squat pyramid up/down steps for 1-10. Dips 50 Abs 50 - Do 50 abs sets until you complete 50 dips - rest with 50 abs as needed **Everything 50** Pullups 50 Squats 50 (135#) Bench press 50 (75-100% of bodyweight) Lunges 25/leg (25-45#) Push Press 50 Leg Press or Dead lift 50 (light) 50 KB swings **SWIM** 50 x 50m - 50 sets of 50m sprints / goal pace sets: 50m free sprint / CSS 50m at goal pace - alternate 25x each.	Pick a fitness test and do it. THEN Run 2 miles Ruck 2 miles Swim 1000m with fins

Winter - Week 3 – Lifting / Non-Impact Cycle

Day 1	Day 2	Day 3
<u>Warmup squat / pushup run pyramid 1-10</u> (25m jogs in between) Bench Press 10,8,6,4,2,1 - work up to 1 rep max BUT rest with 1 min situps and max pullups (weighted) in between each set of bench. Squats 5x5 (front or back) in between squat sets do: - reverse pushups 20 - birds 20 - Arm haulers 20 **Repeat 2-3 times** Dead lift, hang clean - push press complex 5 - 5 - 5 of each exercise non-stop (light weight) <u>Lightweight Shoulders</u> <u>Grip Workout</u> Swim 500m warmup 500-1000m swim with fins Treading 5 minutes no hands without fins. Dynamic Stretches 5 minutes	Cardio <u>20 min bike Pyramid</u> - each minute is tougher than previous minute. 20 min run or longer if you prefer. 5 min tread without hands 1500m swim with fins Upper Core Spread throughout workout: **Repeat 3 times** - Rev. pushups 20 - Birds 20 - Arm Haulers - Plank Pose 1 min <u>Lower back plan - do it later in the evening</u>	<u>Warmup squat / pushup run pyramid 1-10</u> (25m jogs) **Repeat 4-5 times** Pullups max Pulldowns 10 Bench Press 5 Plank pose 1 min Pushups 25 **Repeat 5 times** Squats max 1 min (air or 95lbs) Bear crawls 25m Dips max Situps 1 min Bear crawls 25m Run 2 miles or bike / elliptical 20 minutes Swim 500m warmup **Repeat 5 times** 200m fast - any stroke rest with tread, bounce, float 1 min each set.

Winter - Week 3 – Lifting / Non-Impact Cycle		
Day 4	Day 5	Day 6
Cardio / Core 20 min bike Pyramid - each minute is tougher than previous minute. 20 min run or longer if you prefer. or replace with 30 min ruck 5 min tread without hands 1500m swim with fins Throughout cardio events - stop and do a set of abs / plank pose. Lower back plan - do it later in the evening	Warmup squat / pushup run pyramid 1-10 **Repeat 5 times** Bench Press BW* max reps Pullups *wt - 5 Situps 1 min plank pose 1 min BW -bodyweight* **Repeat 3 times** Squats 5 Dead lift 5 Hang Clean 5 Push Press 5 Bike Pyramid 20 minutes CSS or FREE - 500m timed swim - TEST. Tread water 10 min All dynamic stretches done on land - do in chest deep water / stretch / foam roll..	Run - Ruck - SWIM 2 mile run or 2 mile ruck 1 mile swim with fins OR 25 minute bike or elliptical pyramid. Dynamic Stretches 10 minutes on land or in pool if you choose to swim. Upper Core Spread throughout workout: **Repeat 3 times** - Rev. pushups 20 - Birds 20 - Arm Haulers - Plank Pose 1 min Lower back plan - do it later in the evening

Winter - Week 4 – Lifting / Non-Impact Cycle		
Day 1	Day 2	Day 3
Warmup with **Burpee Pyramid 1-5 (run 25m)** Bench 135# max Situps 1 min Pullups with wt - max Stair crawl up/down or bear crawl 50m **Burpee Pyramid 6-10 (run 25m)** Bench BW max reps Situps 1 min Pullups with wt - max Stair crawl up/down or bear crawl 50m **Burpee Pyramid 11-15 (run 25m)** Bench - 5 of 80% 1RM Situps 1 min Pullups with wt - max Stair crawl up/down or bear crawl 50m Swim 500m warmup 1000m swim with fins Treading 10 minutes no hands without fins. Dynamic Stretches 10 min in water	Warmup squat / run pyramid 1-10 **Repeat 5 times** Squats 5 Dead lift 5 Hang Clean 5 Walk up/down flt of steps 3 times with 45# wt (plate or db) Bike or run 5 min 500m warmup swim without weights 1500m swim with fins OR run or ruck for 30 minutes Lower back plan - do it later in the evening	**Warmup with 15 minutes of Death By Pushups**: Stay in Pushup position for 15 minutes doing 10 pushups every min on the minute. **Repeat 4 times** Pullups wt - max DB rows 10/arm heavy Bench 5 then Pushups max Dips max Situps 1 min Stair crawl up/down Run or bike 15 min **Repeat 3 times** (throughout the workout) - Rev. pushups 20 - Birds 20 - Arm Haulers - Plank Pose 1 min Swim 500m warmup **Repeat 4 times** 250m fast - any stroke rest with tread, bounce, float 1 min each set.

Winter - Week 4 – Lifting / Non-Impact Cycle		
Day 4	Day 5	Day 6
Warmup 10 minutes bike / elliptical Stretch / Foam roll **Repeat 5 times** 5 min run or bike or elliptical or row 5 min stretch and foam roll Swim 15 minutes for max distance -_____ Tread water 5 minutes Do dynamic stretches in pool – chest deep water 5 minutes. (butt kickers, leg swings, Frankenstein kicks, etc..) Lower back plan - do it later in the evening	Warmup pushup / Squat run pyramid 1-10 **Repeat 3 times** Pullups max wt Bench Press 5 Squats 5 Run or bike 5 min intervals **Repeat 3 times** Hang Clean 5 Dead lift 5 Push Press 5 Plank pose 1 min / Stretch 15 min bike, elliptical or run CSS or FREE - 500m timed swim - TEST. Tread water 10 min All dynamic stretches done on land - do in chest deep water / stretch / foam roll..	**Run - Ruck - SWIM** 2 mile run and / or 2 mile ruck 2 mile swim with fins OR 25 minute bike or elliptical pyramid or another 2 mile run. Lower back plan - do it later in the evening

Closing Remarks
Lose the Body Fat / Inches

As we age, gaining weight gets way too easy. Body fat measurement testing requires all military and law enforcement personnel to weigh in and have their height measured. When out of height/weight standards, body fat is measured using the circumference test – measuring the neck and waist or body fat devices.

For starters, if you want to reduce inches that quickly – drink more water. Water retention maybe one of the culprits to your waist size. If you think you may be retaining water, try adding up to a gallon of water a day and you could lose about five to ten pounds of retained water in a few short days. I have seen people lose up to twenty in a week by ONLY adding water to their diet. But once that is done you need to focus on the principles of healthy weight loss below that will help you with your goal:

1) **Eating plan** - This eating plan will help your body keep the metabolism high and burn calories throughout the day. Limiting calories of processed sugar and other processed foods, adding fiber, and adding protein will help lean you out quickly and in a healthy manner.

2) **Cardio workouts** - 4-5 times a week of 45-60 minutes of cardio exercises - elliptical gliding, walking, jogging, swimming, rowing, or biking are great examples of how to burn calories. If you are overweight and need to lose over 50 lbs I do not recommend running. Select a non-impact form of the aerobics listed above.

3) **Muscle training** - Weights or PT program - Lift weights or PT (pushups, situps, pullups, squats, lunges, crunches) every other day 3 times a week or daily with split routines. Building muscle mass will help you also increase metabolism and burn more calories while at rest through the day as well as through your workouts.

4) **Add Water – Eliminate Soda** – You will find that eliminating or reducing sodas, sweet tea / juices in your day and replacing with water will help you quickly lose weight (fat).

See Links: Nutrition | ABDs of Nutrition | Lean Down

Open Invitation - FREE Workouts!

We do local training for FREE in the Annapolis / Severna Park MD area year-round. Our weekly schedule can be found at the Heroes of Tomorrow page. Check in with us prior to attending and fill out the questionnaire on the page above.

If you find this book helpful, let others know. You can also purchase multiple copies at a reduced price from our printer service if you have a large group of people who would benefit from this information. For any info on bulk purchases contact us at the email listed below for price savings per multi-book purchase.

ONLINE COACHING

Also, if you need personal training help, check out the StewSmithFitness.com website where you can train with me through the Online Coaching program.

GOOD LUCK

Thanks for choosing a profession of serving your country and community. It is an honorable profession that requires commitment to stay fit and healthy so you can best perform your duties, to stay alive, and keep others alive.

Good luck with the program and remember to consult your physician first before starting any program if you have not exercised in several months or years. If you need help with any fitness related questions please feel free to email me.

Contact us at stew@stewsmith.com if you need to ask questions about training, this specific workout, or you would like to attend our local workouts, make bulk purchases, or considering online coaching.

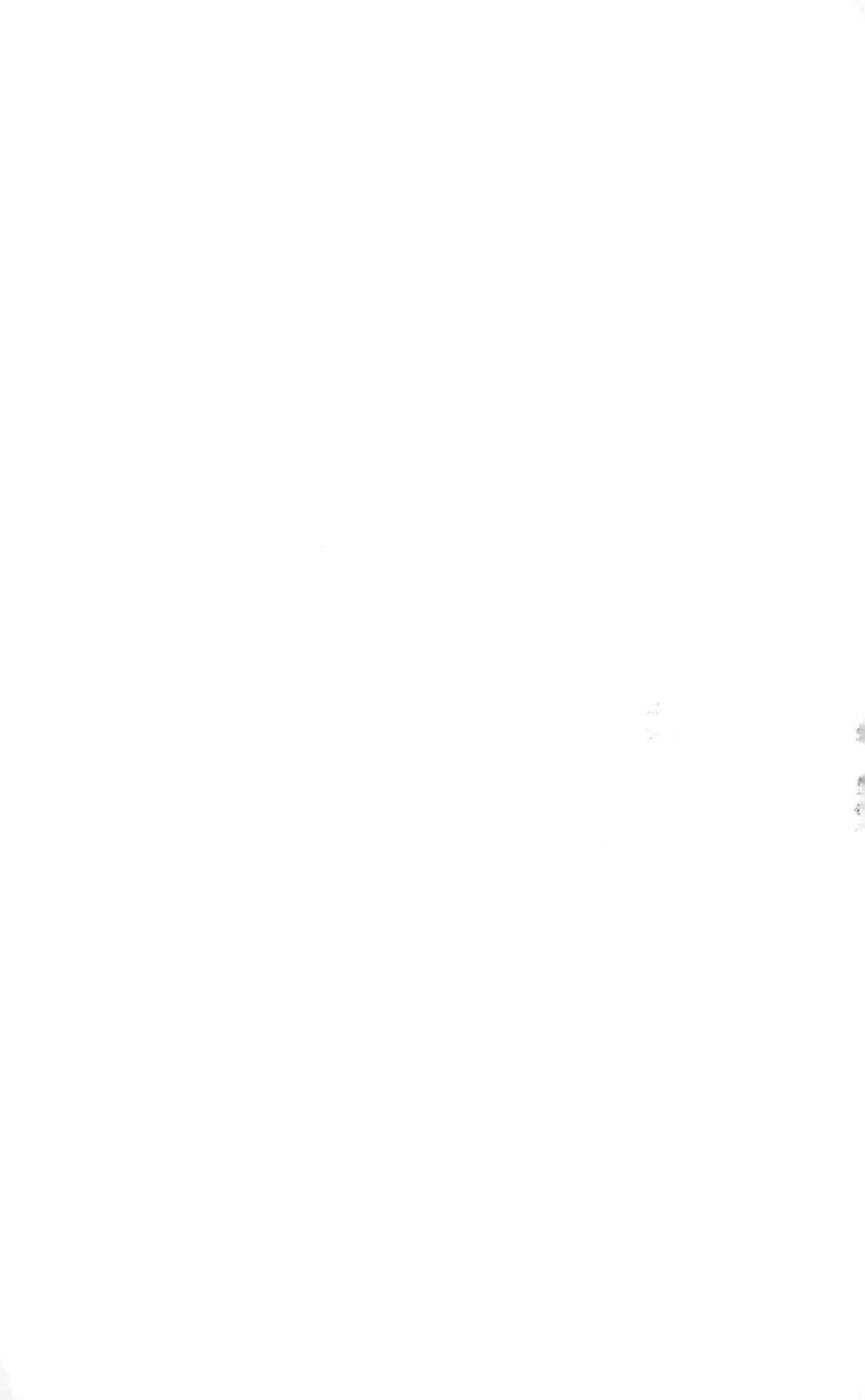

Printed in Great Britain
by Amazon